7 HABITS FOR LIFE

Angela M. Bryan, MPA, RD, LDN

This book contains the opinions and ideas of its author. It is intended to provide helpful and general information on the subjects addressed. It is not in any way a substitute for the advice of the reader's own health care and/or medical professionals. The reader should consult a competent health-care professional and/or physician if the reader needs personal medical, health, dietary, exercise or any other assistance or advice regarding their well-being. The author and publisher specifically disclaim all responsibility for injury, damage, or loss that may incur as a direct or indirect consequence of following any directions or suggestions given in this book.

CONTENTS

A NOTE FROM THE AUTHOR

Unless you live in a bubble, you will eventually get infected with any number of infectious diseases, like the common cold, the flu (influenza), variants of the coronavirus, stomach flu (gastroenteritis), respiratory syncytial virus (RSV), and strep throat. It's just a matter of time. In this book, you will learn 7 habits that have been scientifically proven to strengthen the immune system. Learn the habits. Practice developing them to get ready for what might well be the fight of your life, *for* your life.

HABIT #1
EAT TO LIVE

"To eat is a necessity, but to eat intelligently is an art."
- François de la Rochefoucauld

Fruits and Vegetables: Immunity Protectors!

Researchers split 83 volunteers between ages 65 and 85 into two groups to test their theory that inadequate nutrition could explain why immunity declines as you age. One group ate less than 3 servings of fruits and vegetables a day, while the other group ate at least 5 servings. All were vaccinated against pneumonia. The group that ate 5 or more servings of fruits and vegetables had an 82% better response to the vaccine and this was only after a few months of eating extra servings of fruits and vegetables. [1]

A plant-rich diet will strengthen your immune system [2-7] by providing your body with lots of different antioxidants. [10] Antioxidants protect your immune system from being damaged and encourage the production of white blood cells to protect your body against disease and infection. Fruits and vegetables are packed with a variety of antioxidants such as beta-carotene (dark-green leafy vegetables, sweet potatoes, carrots), vitamin C (citrus fruits, strawberries, bell peppers, mangoes), and vitamin E (nuts, seeds, spinach, broccoli) which boost your immune system. Antioxidants are also found in beans, peas and lentils, which are considered sub-groups of vegetables. You can tell by the rainbow of colors they offer such as black beans, white navy beans, green split peas, red kidney beans, tan black-eyed peas, yellow split peas, pink pinto beans and red lentils. Fresh and dried herbs such as mint, basil, thyme, oregano, rosemary and marjoram, and spices such as turmeric and cinnamon are also rich in antioxidants and give wonderful flavor to food. [8-9]

A nut is actually a dry fruit inside a hard shell. Nuts contain antioxidants called omega-3 fats. Those fats are considered 'essential' because your body can't make them—you have to get them from your diet. Walnuts are packed to the brim with omega-3 fats. Since plants grow from seeds, you shouldn't be surprised to know that they too contain omega-3 fats. Flaxseeds and chia seeds are rich sources. Zinc is a mineral which also helps boost your immune system. Sources are nuts, pumpkin seeds, sesame seeds, beans, and lentils.

Think of yourself as being an artist and your plate or bowl is a blank canvas. 'Paint' with lots of color by filling them with a wide variety of fruits and vegetables every time you eat. The more color you add—green, yellow, black, orange, purple, white, red—the more nutrient-dense that meal will be. Make it cheerful and visually appealing. Each color has something different to offer.

'Paint' For Your Plate And Bowl

BLACK	blackberries, flaxseeds, black beans, kalamata olives, black olives, black plums
PURPLE/ BLUE	blueberries, purple plums, eggplant, figs, purple potatoes, acai, black currants, purple cabbage, red onions, purple kale, raisins, prunes, black grapes, red leaf lettuce, purple carrots
DARK GREEN	*kale, *collards, *salad greens, green olives, broccoli, *mustard greens, parsley, *spinach, cilantro, green beans, *green bell peppers, *turnip greens, mint, basil, thyme, chives, spring onions
LIGHT/ MEDIUM GREEN	*cabbage, celery, granny smith apples, asparagus, okra, kiwi, *limes, pistachios, green olives, chives rosemary, brussels sprout, bok choy, zucchini, green tomatoes
RED/PINK	red lentils, *tomatoes, beets, *strawberries, kidney beans, red small beans, raspberries, rhubarb, red plums, *cranberries, *red bell peppers, watermelon, red delicious apples, *pink grapefruit, pinto beans

BROWN/ TAN	walnuts, pecans, almonds, cashews, macadamias, Brazil nuts
ORANGE	carrots, *papaya, sweet potatoes, *oranges, butternut squash, pumpkin, apricots, persimmon, acorn squash, *orange bell peppers, kumquat, star fruit, peaches, nectarines, cantaloupe
YELLOW	Yellow split peas, *yellow peppers, *mangoes, *lemons, banana peppers, pomelo, golden kiwi, pineapple, turmeric, *grapefruit, yellow figs, yellow apples, yellow watermelon, yellow carrots
WHITE/TAN	bananas, jicama, coconut, black-eyed peas, lychees, soybeans, parsnips, rutabaga, garlic, onions, button mushrooms, navy beans, lotus root, cherimoya, celery root, cauliflower

* Rich in vitamin C—a very powerful antioxidant. Eat at least 4 servings a day.

Some Ideas To Get You Started

Swap and add: The next time you go shopping, take a look at your cart. If you see only 1 color, such as green apples, celery, green bell peppers and frozen broccoli florets (my personal favorite), go back and swap or add more color. For example, add a red bell pepper, swap the apples for red delicious, add sweet potatoes or carrots (but keep the broccoli!)

Make frozen veggie cubes: Puree steamed vegetables. Transfer to ice cube tray. Pop frozen cubes in large freezer bags and label. Use to thicken soups and sauces

Side dishes: Think of vegetables as sides. Include 3 with your dinner meal.

Pile and flip: Vegetables are not just for omelets, scrambling, and frittatas. Like fried eggs? Wait till whites are set, pile on veggies and flip. Pile on more veggies and serve.

Think "what would Chipotle do?': Make sofrito with lots of onion and bell peppers. Pile it on your beans.

Move over gravy: Let sofrito permanently replace your gravy.

Tilt the scale: Make the portion of vegetables in scrambled tofu, omelets, and frittatas much larger than the protein.

Make the dish fit the name: A 'veggie dish' should have lots of colorful vegetables. If not, change the name.

Make frozen bean cubes: Add leftover cooked beans and a little water to a food processor. Blend until a thin paste. Pour into ice cube tray. Transfer frozen cubes to freezer bags and label. Use to thicken soups and sauces.

Add a flavor boost: Add dried or fresh fruit to your salad greens such as blueberries, chopped dates, strawberries, raisins or chopped prunes.

Liven up side dishes: Stir-fry onions, bell peppers and garlic with a fresh herb such as thyme, cilantro, or parsley.

Pile it on plantains, boiled green bananas, sweet potatoes, and cassava (yuca) before serving.

Think differently: Think of onions and fresh garlic as vegetables not as seasonings. Add way more when cooking foods such as beans.

Make chunky vegetable and protein salads: Mix vegetables in egg salad, salmon salad, chicken salad, garbanzo bean salad, tofu salad, such as shredded carrots, chopped purple onions, chopped cucumber, diced tomato, chopped fresh parsley—the options are endless.

Pile and wrap: Pile on the vegetables when making wraps, burritos, and tacos for breakfast—baby spinach, yellow banana peppers, red tomatoes, sliced cucumbers, shredded carrots, the options are endless.

Veggie-up guacamole: Make a chunky guacamole with 1 chopped avocado, 1 chopped tomato, ½ red onion chopped, 1 handful fresh cilantro chopped, juice of 1 lime, ¼ teaspoon cumin, and salt to taste.

Get crunchy: Sprinkle walnuts, slivered almonds, pecans, or pumpkin seeds on your salads and cereal, or use as a topper for muffins, pancakes and quick breads.

Think, "what would Subway do?": You can get at least 9 different vegetables on your sandwich or salad at Subway, including cucumbers, green peppers, lettuce, red onions, baby spinach, tomatoes, banana peppers, and black olives.

Dip it: Baby carrots with roasted red pepper hummus, apple slices or celery sticks with peanut butter, and cucumber slices or bell pepper strips with ranch dressing.

Keep it interesting: Steam, grill, blanch, sauté, broil, stir-fry, and roast.

Don't give up: As they say, it takes at least 21 days to form a new habit.

Buy frozen vegetables: Some people don't buy frozen vegetables because they think that fresh is always best. Actually, they're wrong. Frozen vegetables are processed at the peak of ripeness so their nutrient content is high. Plus, some vegetables tend to wilt rather quickly if they're not eaten within a few days, such as carrots and fresh broccoli. Frozen spinach works best for dips because cooked fresh spinach produces a lot of water which needs to be squeezed out. Frozen broccoli florets steam perfectly in the microwave, retain their bright green color and have a slight sweetness when they're done. I nuke ½ pound of frozen broccoli florets for 5 minutes, drizzle with extra virgin olive oil and eat with breakfast every single morning.

Buy frozen berries: Keep a bag or two in your freezer for adding to smoothies, muffins, pancakes, and making kids' fruit and veggie popsicles. Wild blueberries are my absolute must have. I eat at least 1 cup every day.

Breakfast And Brunch Veggie Ideas
- ✓ Mixed vegetable pancakes
- ✓ Sweet potato and kale hashbrowns
- ✓ Veggie omelets with plantains
- ✓ Avocado, spinach and pineapple smoothie
- ✓ Carrot and mango muffins
- ✓ Marinated grilled tofu and sofrito wrap
- ✓ Mediterranean breakfast burrito
- ✓ Three peppers and onion scrambler
- ✓ Broccoli Normandy fritters
- ✓ Vegetable breakfast tacos
- ✓ Kale, blueberries and pineapple smoothie
- ✓ Tofu or egg sandwich with baby spinach and sliced tomato
- ✓ Spinach banana muffins
- ✓ Savory oatmeal with portabella mushrooms, spinach and sundried tomatoes

These breakfast ideas are not just for weekend eating. A batch of muffins, vegetable pancakes or fritters can be made in advanced. For easy grab-and-go in the morning, just divide into individual portion sizes before placing in quart-sized freezer bags.

I have a friend who can't cook. He orders out for all his meals. However, he's very health conscious and absolutely loves to eat vegetables. Can't get enough of them. I have another friend who can cook and makes the most delicious pancit (a Filipino noodle dish). My mouth is watering right now at the memory. She actually takes the time to cut-up every single vegetable by hand. It's a labor of self-sacrificing love because you'd never know how much she really detests (a far stronger word than hate) cooking! So, I thought of them while writing this section and decided that I must include some vegetable ideas which would be quick and easy for them to whip up.

Vegetable Ideas For People Who Don't Cook Or Detest Cooking

✓ Keep pantry stocked with the following: pop-open canned black beans, a bag of raw, shelled walnuts, a bag of raw shelled pumpkin seeds, small cans of pop-open, sliced black olives, a jar of sliced banana peppers (refrigerate after opening), 1 bottle of extra virgin olive oil for drizzling over veggies and beans, and dried fruits such as golden raisins, cranberries, chopped prunes.

✓ Keep these seasonings and dried herbs in your cupboard: onion powder, garlic powder, cayenne pepper, turmeric, basil, thyme, and oregano. Sprinkle on your veggies for added flavor.

✓ Buy 10 oz. bags of <u>plain</u>, steamable frozen vegetables. Nuke for 4-5 minutes, then drizzle with extra virgin olive oil to taste.

✓ Keep freezer stocked with bags of plain frozen vegetables which have lots of color. Here are some examples from a popular grocery chain in Florida: California blend (broccoli, cauliflower, carrots); Italian blend (cauliflower, lima beans, Italian green beans, carrots); Japanese blend (broccoli, green beans, red peppers, mushrooms); Roma blend (carrots, cauliflower, green beans, sliced zucchini, baby lima beans). Add portion to bowl. Drizzle with extra virgin olive oil. Shake on seasonings. Nuke. Salt to taste.

✓ Keep freezer stocked with bags of frozen dark green leafy vegetables for smoothies, such as collards, spinach, turnip greens, kale, mustard greens.

✓ Keep freezer stocked with frozen berries for smoothies.

✔ Peel ripe bananas, throw away skin. Place in freezer bags for smoothies.

✔ Make a large vegetable and fruit smoothie daily for breakfast. Check out 23 flavor combinations in the next section.

✔ Keep these in your fridge: Large container of store-bought fresh salsa, individually-portioned store-bought guacamole, and shredded carrots.

✔ Make no-cooking-necessary, seasoned black beans. Pop open lid. Dump contents in a glass bowl. Add a generous amount of fresh salsa. Stir. Nuke.

✔ Make haystacks. Spread your favorite tortilla chips on a plate—add the seasoned black beans—now add dark salad greens, yellow banana peppers, sliced black olives, shredded carrots, a generous amount of fresh salsa and add guacamole.

✔ Change up your haystacks. Swap the tortilla chips for dark salad greens and swap the yellow banana peppers for yellow corn. Use frozen corn instead of canned.

✔ Add a few sweet notes such as golden raisins or dried cranberries to haystacks

✔ Make a burrito bowl. Start with seasoned black beans, add yellow corn, shredded carrots, lots of fresh salsa, jalapeno peppers, and guacamole.

✓ Make tacos: Buy the shells. Add your seasoned black beans, top with fresh salsa and guacamole.

✓ Order a large salad and split into sides for 3-4 meals.

✓ Add 2 or more veggie sides to your lunch and dinner order.

✓ Order from Chipotle or similar eateries with lots of vegetable options.

✓ Order vegetable pizza—with extra veggies. Divide portions in freezer bags for quick heat and eat sides.

✓ Cut up leftover vegetable pizza and toss on salads instead of using croutons.

✓ Make Subway a go-to, order-from spot. Tell them you want all of the veggies!

Ideas For Getting Kids To Eat More Fruits And Vegetables

Keep fresh fruits on the kitchen counter. Kids ask for what they see.

Be a positive role model. Seeing you eating and enjoying fruits and vegetables is one of the best ways to get kids to eat more of them.

Replace cookies and chips with fruits and vegetables for snacks.

Take your kids to the local farmers' market or farm near you. Teach them about the foods that are grown in your area.

Let them dip apple wedges and celery sticks in peanut butter, baby carrots in spinach dip or roasted red pepper humus, or cucumber slices and zucchini sticks in ranch dressing. Kids love to dip because it's fun!

Make vegetable and fruit popsicles: It's a frozen smoothie on a stick! Depending on your freezer space, you can make a variety, place them in freezer bags and label. Let kids have them on a lazy breakfast morning when no one is in a rush to head to school or work, as a dessert after dinner. Let them replace the cookies and chips. Remember to change it up— you want kids to get a variety of different vegetables in their diet. Color, color, color. Keep your freezer stocked with frozen green vegetables such as broccoli, turnip greens, spinach, collards, mustard greens and kale. I think your kids will love them! Here are 23 flavor combos to try:

- ✓ Zucchini, mango, banana
- ✓ Avocado, pineapple, banana
- ✓ Cucumber, honeydew, banana
- ✓ Kale, oranges, banana
- ✓ Beets, strawberries, banana
- ✓ Yellow squash, blueberries, banana

- ✓ Turnip greens, mango, banana
- ✓ Collards, honeydew, banana
- ✓ Pumpkin, pineapple, banana
- ✓ Acorn squash, passion fruit, banana
- ✓ Kale, honeydew, banana
- ✓ Spinach, tangerines, banana
- ✓ Cabbage, pineapple, banana
- ✓ Yellow squash, nectarine, banana
- ✓ Kale, cantaloupe, banana
- ✓ Beets, pineapple, banana
- ✓ Pumpkin, cantaloupe, banana
- ✓ Avocado, peach, banana
- ✓ Zucchini, honeydew, banana
- ✓ Mustard greens, pineapple, banana
- ✓ Avocado, mango, banana
- ✓ Spinach, pineapple, banana
- ✓ Collards, blueberries, banana
- ✓ Cucumber, cantaloupe, banana

RETHINK YOUR DRINK

Research now shows, drinking 75-100 grams a day of a sugary solution can weaken your immunity for several hours. The suppression of your immune system starts as soon as 30 minutes after you drink it and can last up to five hours.

Too Much Sugar: Immunity Weakener!

The leading source of added sugars in the American diet doesn't come from cakes, cookies, candy or sweetened cereals—it comes from sugary drinks or sugar-sweetened beverages. [3, 4] The types of sugars added can vary, such as sucrose, raw sugar, malt syrup, high-fructose corn syrup, honey, dextrose, fructose, glucose, corn sweetener, corn syrup, molasses, maltose, and brown sugar. [4] Examples include regular sodas, sports drinks, energy drinks, flavored juice drinks, lemonade, coffee and tea beverages with added sugar, electrolyte replacement drinks, and sweetened water. When you consume too much sugar, it will weaken your immune system. [1, 2] In fact, research now shows that drinking 75-100 grams a day of a sugary solution can weaken your immunity. The suppression of your immune system starts as soon as 30 minutes after you drink it and can last up to five hours. [2]

What does 75-100 grams of a sugary drink look like? [12-13]

Sugar-sweetened Beverage	Size	Grams of Sugar
Arizona Iced Tea	40 oz	105 g
Coca Cola Classic	24 oz	78 g
Pepsi Cola	24 oz	82 g
Dr. Pepper	24 oz	82 g
Mountain Dew	24 oz	84 g
Sprite	24 oz	76 g
Starbucks Caramel Apple Spice [Juice]	16 oz	71 g
Starbucks Peppermint Hot Chocolate	16 oz	74 g
McDonald's Frappe Mocha	Large	89 g
McDonald's Frappe Caramel	Large	89 g
McDonald's Coca Cola Classic	Large	77 g

Between 2011- and 2014, 63% of youth and 49% of adults were recorded as drinking a sugar-sweetened beverage on any given day, [5, 6], Americans drank 52% of sugar-sweetened beverage calories at home, and 48% away from home. [7]– Too much sugar is also more likely to lead to health problems such as weight gain, obesity, type 2 diabetes, heart disease, kidney disease, non-alcoholic liver disease, cavities, and a type of arthritis called gout. [8-11]

The nutritional label on food and beverages will always list the amount of sugar in grams. Grams are a measurement of weight and a teaspoon is a volume measurement. The weight for a teaspoon of sugar is 4 grams (4.2 grams to be exact). To find out how many teaspoons of sugar (or sugar packets) are in a beverage, simply divide the total number of grams of sugar listed by 4.

Total Sugar 46 g = 11 ½ teaspoons of sugar or 11 ½ sugar packets.

Sugar-sweetened Beverage	Size	Grams of Sugar	Teaspoons of Sugar
Arizona Iced Tea	40 oz	105 g	26 ¼
Coca Cola Classic	24 oz	78 g	19 ½
Pepsi Cola	24 oz	82 g	20 ½
Dr. Pepper	24 oz	82 g	20 ½
Mountain Dew	24 oz	84 g	21
Sprite	24 oz	76 g	19
Starbucks Caramel Apple Spice [Juice]	16 oz	71 g	17 ¾
Starbucks Peppermint Hot Chocolate	16 oz	74 g	18 ½
McDonald's Frappe Mocha	Large	89 g	22 ¼
McDonald's Frappe Caramel	Large	89 g	22 ¼
McDonald's Coca Cola Classic	Large	77 g	19 ¾

I reached out to Dr. Trinoda Radcliffe, who practices General Dentistry at her clinic, Radcliffe Family Dental, LLC, in Gary, IN, and asked her what beverage she would recommend for sipping on to stay hydrated during this pandemic and why? This is what she said, "Water. Sugar plus bacteria in the mouth equals acid which causes tooth decay. Sugary drinks such as Gatorade, flavored waters, pop, or juice that are sipped on throughout the day bathe the teeth in sugar which eventually will create acid. Although saliva acts as a natural buffer it cannot combat the onslaught of continually sipping on sugary drinks throughout the day." —Dr. Radcliffe also said, "Coffee is a highly acidic beverage also, and with added sugar and cream it wreaks havoc on the teeth, especially the tooth structure at the gum line. Those areas are then hard to restore and hard to keep clean because bacteria is always going to want to go where the restoration [was done]." Need more reasons to choose water? I'll give you 28:

Gluten-free

No acesulfame potassium

No red dye #40

No monoglycerides

No corn syrup
Generally recognized as safe
Allergen-free
No carrageenan
No potassium sorbate
No diglycerides
No soy lecithin
No cellulose gum
No sodium hexametaphosphate
No aspartame
No blue dye #1
No brominated vegetable oil
No calories
No high fructose corn syrup
No yellow dye #5
No natural flavors
No sodium benzoate
Non-GMO
No calcium disodium EDTA
No gum arabic
No yellow dye #6
No modified cornstarch
No sodium citrate
No caramel coloring

HABIT #3
STAY HYDRATED

"He That Has Satisfied His Thirst, Turns His Back To The Well."
- Baltazar Gracian

Stay Hydrated: Immunity Protector!

Your body has a very complex system called the lymphatic system and it has many jobs. One of them is transporting a watery substance called lymph fluid throughout your body. [1] Lymph fluid contains infection-fighting lymphocytes (highly specialized white blood cells) and other types of immune cells. [1] Each cell has a very unique and important role to play in defending your body against a foreign invader, —such as producing antibodies, recognizing and removing infection-causing cells, and destroying virus-infected cells and cancer cells. As that fluid is moving through your body it's getting rid of toxins and waste materials, and it's also transporting those infection-fighting immune cells to where they are needed. [1] So, what does that have to do with staying hydrated? The word "lympha" is a Latin word which means water.

[2] Lymph fluid is about 96% water. [1] Being dehydrated weakens your immune system. [4-6] That's only one of the many reasons why it's extremely important to drink water.

Between 2005 and 2010, U.S. youth were recorded as drinking an average of 15 ounces of water a day and between 2011 and 2014, U.S. adults were recorded as drinking an average of 39 ounces of water a day. [7, 8] Among U.S. youth, plain water intake is lower in younger children, non-Hispanic blacks, and Mexican-Americans. [4] Among U.S. adults, plain water intake is lower in older adults, lower-income adults, and those with lower education. [8] U.S. adolescents who drink less water tended to drink less milk, eat less fruits and vegetables, drink more sugar-sweetened beverages, and get less physical activity. [9]

There's really no science whatsoever behind the '8 by 8' rule. The amount of water you need to drink depends on a number of things, such as how active you are, the temperature and climate outdoors, your overall health, medications that you're taking, how much you weigh, etc. For example, if it's a hot and humid day, or you live where it's usually hot and humid, you'll need to drink more water to replace water loss from sweating. If you're doing aerobic exercises such as running, cycling, walking, hiking, jogging, etc., you need to drink water before, during and after working out. You will be losing water not only in your sweat but also in your breath. If you're doing any kind of activity and you are sweating, raise the water bottle to your lips and drink.

Are you wondering if you're drinking enough water? The general rule is to check the color of your urine. If it's light yellow or almost clear, you're getting enough. If it's dark gold, you need to drink up. And remember, water is always the best choice for staying hydrated.

Some Ideas On How To Stay Hydrated

- Just woken up? Drink 16 oz. of water.
- Feeling stressed? Take a sip or two of water.
- Case of sodas in your cart? Swap for water.
- Feel like you need to smoke? Drink some water.
- Just got home from work? Drink 16 oz. of water.
- Water? Don't leave home without it.
- Just finished urinating? Take a sip or two of water.
- Ordered soda at the drive-thru? Change to water at the pickup window.
- Your urine is dark yellow? Drink 16 oz. of water.
- Waiting in line at the self-check-out? Take a sip or two of water.
- Feel like you want to snack? Drink some water.
- On your 15 min break? Take a sip or two of water.

- Getting ready to work out? Drink 16 oz. of water.

- Gallons of sweetened iced tea are in your fridge? Swap for water.

- You see a water fountain? Take a sip or two of water.

- Just got to work? Drink 16 oz. of water.

- Still feel like you need to smoke? Drink more water.

- Exercising? Drink some water.

- Dripping sweat? Drink lots of water.

- Feeling overwhelmed? Take a sip or two of water.

- In a Zoom meeting? Take sips of water.

- Tempted to get a soda? Drink some water.

- You just walked past a water fountain? Go back and sip some water.

- Sodas on your grocery list? Cross it out.

- Watching a movie? Take sips of water.

- Just finished working out? Drink 16 oz. of water.

- Standing in front of the vending machine? Select water.

- Bored? Take a sip or two of water.

- Can't remember to drink water? Set a reminder on your phone to alarm every hour while at work. When it goes off, drink 8 oz. of water.

- Reading this book? Sip on water.

★ Sometimes our bodies confuse thirst for hunger.

HABIT #4
SMOKING?
STOP!

Smoking during pregnancy is the largest preventable cause of abnormal lung development in the unborn child. Risk of childhood wheezing and asthma is high for those children [40-43]. Moms who smoke during pregnancy have a higher risk of delivering a still birth (the baby is born dead), premature birth, a baby born with low birth weight, or a baby that's small for gestational age. [45-50]

Mommy, I Can't Breathe!

She was just a tiny little thing
Scrawny, wrinkled, with paper-thin skin
But she was loved, right?
At least, that's what her mommy said
But… but was she, really, loved?
Slowly—ever so slowly
Like the going-under feeling you get
When you're lying on that cold, hard, unyielding slab
of steel
Counting backwards…
Memories of well wishes and celebrating the good news

Faded into heart-wrenching yearnings
To come to grips with
And make some sense of
What I could only described as being
An indifference, for human life
A senseless death!
That's what it was
I shudder at the thought of how it went
But this, this is what they said…
She placed that tiny, innocent soul—in a darkened room
With heavy drapes securely drawn
No light no sun to penetrate
Nor warmth to warm the frigid cold
Windows closed and sealed so tight
That toxic air could not escape!
Nor fresh air enter
Through the cracks
Or gaps between the windowsill
It was a coffin! Not a room
A shroud of death of pain and certain gloom
No chance to live
Nor see the one
For whom she needed most to care
To lift the heavy load of weight

That pressed

And crushed

And choked the life

From one who did not understand!

Why such an act

A choice from one

Same sex as her

Would choose to do

What mattered not to her own self

But, it did to her

They said…

For 9 long months

She pumped and forced

Those cloudy, grey thick, fumes of smoke

Inside that hot and stuffy chamber

Where that angel lay

Gasping for breath

With none to save those lungs from death

And so, they gave out

Limp and still

Like rag-doll weak

She slumped

And was no more.

- Angela M. Bryan, 11/28/2020

Pregnant and smoking? Stop! Call your doctor. Don't have a doctor? Phone 1-800-QUIT-NOW (1-800-784-8669). This is the number for the American Lung Association's program, *Freedom From Smoking*. That number gives you access to their specially trained counselors in all states. They will help you make a plan. Stick with it and don't give up. No matter how difficult it gets, don't give up on quitting smoking.

Your unborn child's ability to survive may well depend on it.

Smoking? Immunity Weakener!

Smoking greatly weakens your immune system. [1-7] That's why smokers are more likely to get all kinds of infections [8-16, 34-37] including infected gums (periodontal disease). [10-16] Smoking severely worsens the health of the gums. Once damaged, the weakened immune system makes it harder for smokers to fight the infection and heal. [17-19, 22-26] Smokers have at least twice the risk of gum disease compared to non-smokers. [20] The risk increases the longer you smoke and the more cigarettes you smoke.

[21] Since smokers have a weak immune system, treatments for gum disease may not work. [22-26] Tobacco

use in any form—cigarettes, pipes, and spit tobacco—increases your risk for gum disease. [14, 27]

Smoking makes it really hard for your body to heal a wound. [28-33] To help the reader better understand how smoking affects wound healing, I reached out to Dr. Alex Evans, who is a trauma and critical care surgeon. This is what he said, "Smoke and inhalation toxins produced by smoke in cigarettes along with the nicotine by itself, all cause a vasoconstrictor effect on blood vessels. In other words, the blood vessels squeeze shut when you have byproducts of smoke and the active drug nicotine within the blood vessels. When that happens, wounds cannot heal because blood supply does not get to the areas that allow wounds to heal. In order for wounds to heal, they have to have nutrition, oxygen, and the cells that grow new tissue and new skin. This is stopped by lack of blood supply. If there is also no good blood supply, then bacteria can grow in wounds causing wound infections. Wound infections then destroy healing tissue and leave the wound open."

Smokers also get more severe and frequent respiratory tract infections. [34-37] Examples include lung cancer, chronic obstructive pulmonary disease (COPD), interstitial lung diseases and bronchial asthma, which are caused and worsened by smoking [38, 39]. A study done at the

University of Cincinnati, Ohio, showed smoking can cause the body's immune system to attack the lung tissue and cause severe respiratory disorders. [1] The findings were reported in the March 2009 issue of the "Journal of Clinical Investigation".

All tobacco-related illnesses, including asthma, COPD and coronary artery disease are known to reduce lung capacity—the amount of air your lungs can hold, and weaken your immune system. [40]

The Health Benefits of Quitting Smoking over Time [51]

Time After Quitting	Health Benefits
Minutes	Heart rate drops
24 hours	Nicotine level in blood drops to zero
Several days	Carbon monoxide in blood drops to level of someone who does not smoke
1 to 12 months	Coughing and shortness of breath decrease
1 to 2 years	Risk of heart attack drops sharply
3 to 6 years	Added risk of coronary heart disease drops by half
5 to 10 years	Added risk of cancers of mouth, throat and voice box drop by half
5 to 10 years	Risk of stroke decreases

10 years	Added risk of lung cancer drops by half after 10-15 years Risk of cancers of bladder, esophagus, and kidney decrease
15 years	Risk of coronary heart disease is close to that of someone who does not smoke
20 years	Risk of cancers of mouth, throat, voice box and pancreas is close to that of someone who does not smoke.

You really don't want a weakened immune system when you get infected with the coronavirus. Decide to stop smoking today. Call your doctor. Don't have a doctor? Phone 1-800-QUIT-NOW (1-800-784-8669). This is the number for the American Lung Association's program, *Freedom From Smoking.* That number gives you access to their specially trained counselors in all states. They will help you make a plan. Stick with it—don't give up. No matter how difficult it gets, don't give up on quitting smoking.

HABIT #5
SLEEP

"And if tonight my soul may find her peace in sleep, and sink in good oblivion, and in the morning wake like a new-opened flower then I have been dipped again in God, and new-created."
- AD.H. Lawrence

Get Your Zzzzzzs: Immune System Booster!

Studies show that sleep has a powerful effect on the immune system. [1-18, 24] It is associated with a reduced risk for infection and can improve infection outcomes and vaccination responses. [1, 13]

When sleep is restricted or the body is deprived of sleep, it has a negative impact on the immune system. [5-11] Sleep loss is related to a higher risk for infection. [12] A total of 164 healthy men and women volunteered for a study on whether sleep makes it easier for people to catch a cold. Participants were quarantined, given nasal drops that had the cold virus and monitored over 5 days. There was a greater risk of catching a cold after having less than 5 or between 5 to 6 hours of sleep compared to having more than 7 hours of sleep. [15] Those with less than 7 hours of sleep each night were 3 times more likely to develop a cold than those with 8 or more hours. [16] There was more than a 50% decrease in antibodies to the flu vaccine when sleep was restricted to 4 hours a night for 6 days followed by 12 hours a night for 7 days compared to having regular hours of sleep. [17] A modest amount of sleep loss—restricting sleep to 4 hours for 1 night, reduced natural killer cell activity to about 72% compared with those who had a full night's sleep. [18] Your goal should be to improve both the quality and the quantity of your sleep. [21]

Sleep quality refers to how well you sleep at night— how refreshed you feel when you wake up. Most people need 7 to 8 hours of good quality sleep each night.

[22] For adults, that means you usually fall asleep in 30 minutes or less, you sleep soundly through the night with no more than 1 awakening, and drift back off to sleep within 20 minutes. [21] Poor sleep quality is when you have trouble falling and/or staying asleep, and a large portion of your sleep time is spent staring at the ceiling or counting sheep. It leaves you feeling exhausted the next morning.

Healthy People 2020, which outlines the national health goals for the next decade, recommends that adults get 7 or more hours of sleep each day. [19] But, young adults between

18 and 25 years of age, may need as little as 6 hours of sleep per night—and others may require up to 10 or possibly 11 hours to fully restore their energy. [21] Each person is different and you are the best judge in determining whether you feel alert and rested after 7 hours of sleep or if you'd benefit from getting 1 or more hours of shut eye. [21, 22] About 32% of U.S healthcare workers report getting 6 hours or less of sleep each day [23]. That amount is considered to be too short by most sleep experts. [19] One way of estimating how many hours you need to sleep is to take note of the length of time you sleep towards the end of a stress free and relaxing 2-week vacation—when you're not under any time pressures and you can go to bed when you're tired and wake up without an alarm. [25]

Here Are 14 Proven Evidence-Based Tips For Sleeping Better At Night

1. **Increase bright light exposure during the day:** [26-29] Natural sunlight or artificial bright light during the day helps keep your circadian rhythm healthy and improves nighttime sleep quality and duration. [26-29]

2. **Reduce blue light exposure in the evening:** [30-34] Electronics such as smart phones, tablets,

computers, and laptops emit large amounts of blue light. Blue light effects your circadian rhythm, tricking your brain to think that it's still daytime. This reduces your melatonin level which is important for helping you to relax and get deep sleep. Fluorescent lights and LED lights also emit blue lights. Here are ways to limit your exposure to blue light at night.

- ✓ Wear blue light blocking glasses.
- ✓ Download a blue light filter app to your PC such as f.lux.
- ✓ Install an app that blocks blue light on your smartphone.
- ✓ Stop watching TV and turn off any bright lights 2 hours before heading to bed.
- ✓ If you're using Microsoft Windows 10, there's no need to download any additional software. Microsoft added a 'Blue Light' filter known as Night light. To enable: Select Start>Settings>System>Display>Night light>Night light settings.

3. **Limit irregular or long daytime naps**: Taking long naps may impair sleep quality. If you take regular naps and sleep well, continue. If you have

trouble sleeping at night stop napping or shorten your daytime naps to a power nap of 20-30 minutes. [35-39]

4. **Sleep and wake up at consistent times:** Get in the habit of waking up and going to bed at similar times—especially on the weekends. Irregular sleep patterns can alter your circadian rhythm and melatonin level which signal your body to sleep. After several weeks, you may not even need an alarm. [40-43]

5. **Don't drink alcohol:** [44-49] Drinking alcohol before bed can reduce nighttime melatonin production and lead to disrupted sleep patterns. [44-49]

6. **Create a room for sleeping:** [50-53] Make sure your bedroom is a relaxing, clean, quiet, and enjoyable place for sleeping.

7. **Set your bedroom temperature**: [54-58] Set different temperatures to see what's most comfortable for you. Around 70°F (20°C) seems to work best for most people.

8. **Don't eat dinner late in the evening:** [59-63] Eating large meals before bed can lead to poor sleep and hormone disruption.

9. **Take a relaxing shower or bath:** [64-68] A warm bath, shower, or foot bath before bed can help you relax and improve your quality of sleep.

10. **Relax and clear your mind**: [69-72] Relaxation techniques before bed, including meditation, deep breathing, and hot baths, may help you to fall asleep.

11. **Rule out a sleep disorder:** [73-77] Poor sleep is sometimes due to a health condition, such as sleep apnea. Contact your healthcare provider if poor sleep is a consistent problem.

12. **Get comfortable bedding**: [78-83] Your bed, mattress, and pillow greatly affect sleep quality, and potential joint or back pain. Buy a new mattress every 5-8 years. Try to buy the highest quality you can afford. This could be an expensive quick fix to getting quality sleep— especially if it's been several years since you bought new bedding.

13. **Exercise regularly—but not before bedtime:** [84-89] Regular exercise during daylight is one of the best ways for getting a good night's sleep. On the flip side, exercising too late in the day may cause sleep problems. In people with severe insomnia, exercise offered more benefits than most drugs. Exercise reduced the amount of time to fall asleep by

55%, total night wakefulness by 30%, and anxiety by 15%, while increasing total sleep time by 18%. [89]

14. **Don't drink any liquids before bed:** [90-91] Excessive urinating during the night affects sleep quality. Try not to drink any liquids 1-2 hours before going to bed. Use the bathroom right before going to bed.

HABIT #6
GET YOUR EX
BACK

"The only exercise that some people get, is jumping to conclusions, running down their friends, side-stepping responsibility, and pushing their luck."
- Author Unknown

Exercise: Every Step is Powerful Medicine!

The COVID-19 pandemic placed a damper on a whole lot of things we used to do to keep fit and stay in shape. Gyms were closed to help slow down the spread of the virus and get people to social distance. You may have missed the fun that comes from hiking with a group or walking with a friend. With the challenges that working from home and being quarantined brought, you may have even lacked the motivation to continue or even start a routine on your own. Working from home also led us to doing a lot more sitting down and far less movement than we did before the pandemic—and it shows on our belly, around our waist and hips, and definitely on the bathroom scale. It crept up on us since we hardly got 'dressed' to go anywhere—pajamas were our work wear, and sweats did just fine for most anything else. To add more fuel to the fire, if you're like thousands of Americans who are out of work and having a hard time finding money to pay rent and put food on the table, exercise might be quite low on your to-do list. Well, hopefully, this chapter will motivate you to get your Ex back—and this time, keep it.

Exercise is powerful medicine for the body. [1-26] It makes your immune system stronger. [1-8] It helps you get a better night's sleep (quality sleep). [9-12] It improves blood sugar control in type 2 diabetes. [13-16] It helps control high blood pressure. [17-20] It's great for your mental health and reduces stress. [21-26] Exercise has been used as 'medicine' to help treat 26 different diseases: psychiatric diseases (depression, anxiety, stress, schizophrenia); neurological diseases (dementia, Parkinson's disease, multiple sclerosis); metabolic diseases (obesity, hyperlipidemia, metabolic syndrome, polycystic ovarian syndrome, type 2 diabetes, type 1 diabetes); cardiovascular diseases (hypertension, coronary heart disease, heart failure, cerebral apoplexy, and claudication intermittent); pulmonary diseases (chronic obstructive pulmonary disease, asthma, cystic fibrosis);

musculo-skeletal disorders (osteoarthritis, osteoporosis, back pain, rheumatoid arthritis); and cancer. [17, 19]

Since this book will be read by people in different age groups and fitness levels, I wanted to include an exercise idea that would be suitable for most people. So, I immediately thought of my sister Donna who is a physical therapist and has been practicing for over 30 years, and this is what she said, "walking is the best exercise as it needs no special skill or equipment." Walking is budget-friendly since most people already own a pair or two of sneakers, so there's little or no cost to start. Walking is much easier on knees and joints than running or jogging. You can move at your own pace—a casual stroll, brisk walking or power walking with arms bent and quicker, shorter steps. You can plan your walk when it suits you best. If you're an early bird like me, you might like walking in the morning to start your day off on the right foot. You can go for a casual or brisk walk at lunch or break time. You could even do a lap or two around the parking lot at the grocery store before heading inside. There are so many types of walking with different speed variations such as the casual stroll, brisk walking, power walking, race walking, Nordic walking, and marathon walking. I also asked Donna for exercise ideas for nursing home residents—for people who are chair-or bed-bound. This is what she said, "There are also several videos on chair exercises … basically move as much of your body as you can as often as you can whether chair-bound or bed-bound."

Most people can safely take walks as an exercise, but first check with your doctor if you have a health problem or if any part of your body has been hurt. Also check with your doctor first if it's been a long time since you've been active or if you're very overweight.

HABIT #7
LAUGH

"A smile starts on the lips, a grin spreads to the eyes, a chuckle comes from the belly; but a good laugh bursts forth from the soul, overflows, and bubbles all around. "
— Carolyn Birmingham

Laughter: Immune System Booster!

It's true, a merry heart does one good just as medicine does. Research shows that laughing boosts and strengthens your immune system. [1-8] It also helps in managing pain by increasing your tolerance for pain [9-12], it reduces stress [13-21], and it improves your mood and makes you feel happy. [22-24]

Here are some quotes from famous doctors: [25]

"The simple truth is that happy people generally don't get sick." — Bernie Siegel, M.D. (an internationally-recognized expert in the field of cancer treatment and complementary holistic medicine)

"The best clinicians understand that there is an intrinsic physiological intervention brought about by positive emotions such as mirthful laughter, optimism and hope." – Lee Berk, DrPH, Assoc. Res. Pro Loma Linda School of Medicine

"For the most part, when you go and get medical treatment, a clinician is not necessarily going to tell you to take two aspirins and watch Laurel and Hardy, but the reality is that's where we are and it's more real than ever. There's a real science to this. And it's as real as taking a drug." – Lee Berk, DrPH, Assoc. Res. Pro Loma Linda School of Medicine

"Daily opportunities for laughter are important for patients with diabetes" – Keiko Hayashi, RN, PhD

"Believe it or not, having a really hearty chuckle can help too. This is because laughing gets the diaphragm moving and this plays a vital part in moving blood around the body." – Dr. Andrea Nelson, University of Leeds School of Healthcare

Start with a smile: If it's been a long time since you laughed—you might want to start with a smile. Do it right now as your read this. Take a deep breath—and as you slowly exhale, put a big, warm smile on your face as if you're eating a warm, freshly-baked chocolate chip cookie. Now, think of something sad, but keep smiling. It's really hard to keep a negative or unhappy thought in your mind while keeping a smile on your face.

Watch stand-up comedians: This is as simple as it gets folks. They get paid to make people laugh. Don't know where to start? Google or ask a friend.

Watch comedies: They're made for one purpose and one purpose only—to make people laugh. You know where to start.

Read and share Knock, Knock Jokes:
Such as these: [26]

- ✓ Knock, Knock! Who's there? Ken. Ken who? Ken I come in? It's cold out here.
- ✓ Knock! Knock! Who's there? Needle. Needle who? Needle little help getting in the door!
- ✓ Knock! Knock! Who's there? Candice. Candice who? Candice door open, or what?
- ✓ Knock! Knock! Who's there? Santa. Santa who? Santa email reminding you I'd be here, and you STILL make me wait in the cold!
- ✓ Knock! Knock! Who's there? Carmen. Carmen who? Carmen let me in already!
- ✓ Knock! Knock! Who's there? Scold. Scold who? Scold outside—let me in!
- ✓ Knock! Knock! Who's there? Otto. Otto who? Otto know what's taking you so long!

✓ Knock! Knock! Who's there? Stopwatch. Stopwatch who? Stopwatch you're doing and pay attention!

✓ Knock! Knock! Who's there? Howl. Howl who? Howl you know if you don't open the door?

✓ Knock! Knock! Who's there? A broken pencil. A broken pencil who? Never mind, it's pointless.

✓ Knock! Knock! Who's there? Owls say. Owls say who? Yes, they do.

✓ Knock! Knock! Who's there? Beets. Beets who? Beets me!

✓ Knock! Knock! Who's there? I am. I am who? You tell me!!

✓ Knock, Knock! Who's there? Cargo! Cargo who? Cargo beep, beep!

✓ Knock, Knock! Who's there? Wire. Wire who? Wire you always asking 'who's there'?

✓ Knock! Knock! Who's there? Mary and Abbey. Mary and Abbey who? Mary Christmas and Abbey New Year!

Here's a Mixture of Laugh Quotes and Quotes about Laughing [27]

Laughter lets me relax. It's the equivalent of taking a deep breath, letting it out and saying, 'This, too, will pass'. - Odette Pollar

Laughter opens the lungs, and opening the lungs ventilates the spirit. - Unknown

Laughter serves as a blocking agent. Like a bulletproof vest, it may help protect you against the ravages of negative emotions that can assault you in disease. - Norman Cousins

Your body cannot heal without play. Your mind cannot heal without laughter. Your soul cannot heal without joy. - Catherine Rippenger Fenwick

Mirth is like a flash of lightning that breaks through a gloom of clouds and glitter for the moment. Cheerfulness keeps up daylight in the mind, filling it with steady and perpetual serenity. - Samuel Johnson

I will follow the upward road today; I will keep my face to the light. I will think high thoughts as I go my way; I will do what I know is right. I will look for the flowers by the side of the road; I will laugh and love and be strong. I will try to lighten another's load this day as I fare along. - Mary S. Edgar

Among those whom I like or admire, I can find no common denominator, but among those whom I love, I can: all of them make me laugh. - W. H. Auden

I have not seen anyone dying of laughter, but I know millions who are dying because they are not laughing. - Dr. Madan Kataria

An optimist laughs to forget; a pessimist forgets to laugh. - Tom Nansbury

And keep a sense of humor. It doesn't mean you have to tell jokes. If you can't think of anything else, when you're my age, take off your clothes and walk in front of a mirror. I guarantee you'll get a laugh. - Art Linkletter

A good laugh is sunshine in the house. - William Thackeray A smile is a curve that sets everything straight. - Phyllis Diller

Grim care, moroseness, and anxiety—all this rust of life ought to be scoured off by the oil of mirth. Mirth is God's medicine. - Henry Ward Beeche

I never would have made it if I could not have laughed. It lifted me momentarily out of this horrible situation, just enough to make it livable. - Viktor Frankl

As soap is to the body, so laughter is to the soul. - A Jewish proverb

Cancer is probably the unfunniest thing in the world, but I'm a comedian, and even cancer couldn't stop me from seeing the humor in what I went through. - Gilda Radner

When you do laugh, open your mouth wide enough for the noise to get out without squealing, throw your head back as though you were going to be shaved, hold on to your false hair with both hands and then laugh till your soul gets thoroughly rested. - Josh Billings

Acknowledgements

Thanks to God—Creator of all life—for giving me the
love of writing, a creative mind, a sense of humor, and the
determination to live a long and healthy life, until such
time that my borrowed breath returns to Him.
Thanks to my late parents, Thomas and Thelma Bryan, for
their love and support throughout the years.
A special thanks to my friends
Dr. Trinoda Radcliffe, D.D.S and
Dr. Alex Evans, M.D
And last, but not least a special thanks to my Irish twin and
beloved sister
Donna Eaton, PT ☺
Unbeknowst to them, all three contributed to the
writing of this book. They took the time out of their
busy schedules to answer my questions. They shared their
professional knowledge and clinical expertise in their
respective fields of health care.
Their contribution was invaluable to the writing of this
book and for that, I am truly grateful.

About the Author

Angela is a registered dietitian/nutritionist and also a licensed dietitian/nutritionist in the state of Florida. She received her bachelor's degree in dietetics from Andrews University in Berrien Springs, MI. She holds a Master's of Public Affairs in Human Services Administration, from Northwest Indiana University. Angela believes in practicing what she preaches—in leading by example. She believes that is the best and most effective way of motivating others to adopt healthier eating habits and life-styles. Angela firmly believes that true wealth is your health and a worthy investment.

INDEX

HABIT # 1: EAT TO LIVE

[1] Gibson A, Edgar J, Neville C, et al. Effect of fruit and vegetable consumption on immune function in older people: a randomized controlled trial. *Am J Clin Nutr.* 2012;96(6):1429-16

[2] Malter M, Schriever G, Eilber U. Natural killer cells, vitamins, and other blood components of vegetarian and omnivorous men. *Nutr Cancer.* 1989;12:271-278;

[3] Carddock JC, Neale EP, People GE, Probst YC. Vegetarian-based dietary patterns and their relation with inflammatory and immune biomarkers: a systematic review and meta-analysis. *Adv Nutr* 2019;10:133 151.

[4] Zhu F, Du B, Xu B. Anti-inflammatory effects of phytochemicals from fruits, vegetables, and food legumes: a review. *Crit Rev Food Sci Nutr.* 2018 May 24;58(8):1260-1270. doi: 10.108010408398.2016.1251390. Epub 2017 Jun 12. PMID: 28605204.

[5]   Soundararajan P, Kim JS. Anti-carcinogenic glucosinolates in cruciferous vegetables and their antagonistic effects on prevention of cancers. *Molecules.* 2018 Nov 15;23(11):2983. doi: 10.3390/molecules23112983. PMID: 30445746; PMCID: PMC6278308.

[6]   Alwarawrah Y, Kiernan K, MacIver NJ. Changes in nutritional status impact immune cell metabolism and function. *Front Immunol.* 2018;9:1055-1069.

[7]   Haddad EH, Berk LS, Kettering JD, Hubbard RW, Peters WR. Dietary intake and biochemical, hematologic, and immune status of vegans compared with nonvegetarians. *Am J Clin Nutr.* 1999;70(3 Suppl):586S-593S.

[8]   Tapsell LC, Hemphill I, Cobiac L, Patch CS, Sullivan DR, Fenech M, Roodenrys S, Keogh JB, Clifton PM, Williams PG, Fazio VA, Inge KE. Health benefits of herbs and spices: the past, the present, the future. *Med J Aust.* 2006 Aug 21;185(S4):S1-S24. PMID: 17022438.

[9]   Jiang TA. Health benefits of culinary herbs and spices. *J AOAC Int.* 2019 Mar 1;102(2):395-411. doi: 10.5740/jaoacint.18-0418. Epub 2019 Jan 16. PMID: 30651162.

[10] Dragsted LO, Pedersen A, Hermetter A, Basu S, Hansen M, Haren GR, Kall M, Breinholt V, Castenmiller JJ, Stagsted J, Jakobsen J, Skibsted L, Rasmussen SE, Loft S, Sandström B. The 6-a-day study: effects of fruit and vegetables on markers of oxidative stress and 7 Habits for Life antioxidative defense in healthy nonsmokers. *Am J Clin Nutr.* 2004 Jun;79(6):1060-72. doi: 10.1093/ajcn/79.6.1060. PMID: 15159237.

HABIT # 2 RETHINK YOUR DRINK

[1] Yu S, Zhang G, Jin LH. A high-sugar diet affects cellular and humoral immune responses in drosophila. *Exp Cell Res.* 2018 Jul 15;368(2):215-224. doi: 10.1016/j. yexcr.2018.04.032. Epub 2018 May 1. PMID: 29727694.

[2] Albert Sanchez, JL, Reeser, HS, Lau, PY, Yahiku, RE, Willard, PJ, McMillan, SY, Cho, AR. Roles of sugar in human neutrophilic phagocytosis. *The American Journal of Clinical Nutrition,* 1973 Nov:26(11):1180-1184.

[3] Centers for Disease Control and Prevention. Get the facts: sugar-sweetened beverages and consumption. Available from: https:///www.cdc.gov

[4] U.S Department of Agriculture, U.S. Department of Health and Human Services. Dietary guidelines for Americans, 2015-2010. 8th edition. Washington DC: U.S. Government Printing Office; 2015.

[5] Rosinger A, Herrick K, Gahche J, Park S. Sugar-sweetened beverage consumption among U.S. youth, 2011–2014. *NCHS Data Brief.* 2017;271. Hyattsville, MD: National Center for Health Statistics.

[6] Rosinger A, Herrick K, Gahche J, Park S. Sugar-sweetened beverage consumption among U.S. adults, 2011–2014. *NCHS Data Brief.* 2017;270. Hyattsville, MD: National Center for Health Statistics.

[7] Kit BK, Fakhouri TH, Park S, Nielsen SJ, Ogden CL. Trends in sugar-sweetened beverage consumption among youth and adults in the United States: 1999-2010. *Am J Clin Nutr.* 2013;98(1):180-188.

[8] Malik VS, Hu FB. Sugar-sweetened beverages and cardiometabolic health: an update of the evidence. *Nutrients.* 2019;11(8):1840.

[9] Malik VS, Hu FB. Fructose and cardiometabolic health: what the evidence from sugar-sweetened beverages tells us. *J Am Coll Cardiol.* 2015;66(14):1615-1624.

[10] Bomback A, Derebail V, Shoham D, et al. Sugar-sweetened soda consumption, hyperuricemia, and kidney disease. *Kidney International.* 2010;77(7):609-616.

[11] Valenzuela MJ, Waterhouse B, Aggarwal VR, Bloor K, Doran T. Effect of sugar-sweetened beverages on oral health: a systematic review and meta-analysis. *Eur J Public Health.* 2020 Aug 23;ckaa147. doi: 10.1093/eurpub/ckaa147. Epub ahead of print. PMID: 32830237.

[12] Starbucks website. Available from: https//www.Starbucks.com

[13] McDonald's Nutrition Calculator. Available from: https://www.mcdonalds.com

HABIT #3: STAY HYDRATED

[1] Gray's Anatomy for Students: With Student Consult Online Access. Drake, R, Vogl, A., Mitchell, A. 2019.

[2] Lymph - definition and more from the Free Merriam-Webster Dictionary. Available from: www.merriam-webster.com.

[3] Chishaki T, Umeda T, Takahashi I, Matsuzaka M, Iwane K, Matsumoto H, Ishibashi G, Ueno Y, Kashiwa N, Nakaji S. Effects of dehydration

on immune functions after a judo practice session.
Luminescence. 2013 Mar-Apr;28(2):114-20.
doi: 10.1002/bio.2349. Epub 2012 Feb 24.
PMID: 22362640.

[4] Guseĭnova ST. Morphological changes in lymphoid
nodules of small intestine in dehydration]. *Morfologiia.*
2010;137(5):44-7. Russian. PMID: 21500432.

[5] Guseinov TS, Guseinova ST. Effect of dehydration on
morphogenesis of the lymphatic network and immune
structures in the small intestine. *Bull Exp Biol Med.*
2008 Jun;145(6):755-7. doi: 10.1007/s10517-008- 0187-
2. PMID: 19110570.

[6] Drewnowski A, Rehm CD, Constant F. Water
and beverage consumption among children age
4-13y in the United States: analyses of 2005-
2010 NHANES data. *Nutr J.* 2013 Jun 19;12:85.
doi: 10.11861475/-2891-12-85. PMID: 23782914;
PMCID: PMC3698018.

[7] Rosinger AY, Herrick KA, Wutich AY, Yoder JS,
Ogden CL. Disparities in plain, tap and bottled water
consumption among US adults: National Health and
Nutrition Examination Survey (NHANES) 2007-
2014. *Public Health Nutr.* 2018 Jun;21(8):1455-1464.

doi: 10.1017/ S1368980017004050. Epub 2018 Feb 1. PMID: 29388529; PMCID: PMC7474465.

[8] Park S, Onufrak S, Cradock A, Patel A, Hecht C, Merlo C, Blanck HM. Correlates of infrequent plain water intake among US high school students: National Youth Risk Behavior Survey, 2017. *Am J Health Promot.* 2020 Jun;34(5):549-554. doi: 10.11770890117120911885/. Epub 2020 Mar 18. PMID: 32186199; PMCID: PMC7546545.

HABIT # 4 SMOKING? STOP!

[1] Hersey P, Prendergast D, Edwards A. Effects of cigarette smoking on the immune system. Follow-up studies in normal subjects after cessation of smoking. *Med J Aust.* 1983 Oct 29;2(9):425-9. PMID: 6633406.

[2] Mehta H, Nazzal K, Sadikot RT. Cigarette smoking and innate immunity. *Inflamm Res.* 2008 Nov;57(11):497-503. doi: 10.1007/s00011-008-8078-6. PMID: 19109742

[3] Qiu F, Liang CL, Liu H, Zeng YQ, Hou S, Huang S, Lai X, Dai Z. Impacts of cigarette smoking on immune responsiveness: up and down or upside down? *Oncotarget.* 2017 Jan 3;8(1):268-284. doi:

10.18632/oncotarget.13613. PMID: 27902485; PMCID: PMC5352117.

[4] Ebihara S, Ebihara T, Okazaki T, Sasaki H. Cigarette smoking, cough reflex, and respiratory tract infection. *Arch Intern Med.* 2005 Apr 11;165(7):814. doi: 10.1001/archinte.165.7.814-a. PMID: 15824305.

[5] Robbins CS, Dawe DE, Goncharova SI, Pouladi MA, Drannik AG, Swirski FK, Cox G, Stämpfli MR. Cigarette smoke decreases pulmonary dendritic cells and impacts antiviral immune responsiveness. *Am J Respir Cell Mol Biol.* 2004 Feb;30(2):202-11. doi: 10.1165/rcmb.2003-0259OC. Epub 2003 Aug 14. PMID: 12920055.

[6] Mehta H, Nazzal K, Sadikot RT. Cigarette smoking and innate immunity. *Inflamm Res.* 2008 Nov;57(11):497-503. doi: 10.1007/s00011-008-8078-6. PMID: 19109742.

[7] Elisia I, Lam V, Cho B, Hay M, Li MY, Yeung M, Bu L, Jia W, Norton N, Lam S, Krystal G. The effect of smoking on chronic inflammation, immune function and blood cell composition. *Sci Rep.* 2020 Nov 10;10(1):19480. doi: 10.1038/s41598-020-76556-7. PMID: 33173057; PMCID: PMC7655856.

[8] Danov O, Wolff M, Bartel S, Böhlen S, Obernolte H, Wronski S, Jonigk D, Hammer B, Kovacevic D, Reuter S, Krauss-Etschmann S, Sewald K. Cigarette smoke affects dendritic cell populations, epithelial barrier function, and the immune response to viral infection with H1N1. *Front Med (Lausanne).* 2020 Nov 6;7:571003. doi: 10.3389/fmed.2020.571003. PMID: 33240904; PMCID: PMC7678748.

[9] L, Benowitz NL. Cigarette smoking and infection. *Arch Intern Med.* 2004 Nov 8;164(20):2206-16. doi: 10.1001/archinte.164.20.2206. PMID: 15534156.

[10] Zee KY. Smoking and periodontal disease. *Aust Dent J.* 2009 Sep;54;Suppl 1:S44-50. doi: 10.1111/j.1834-7819.2009.01142.x. PMID: 19737267.

[11] Bergström J. Tobacco smoking and chronic destructive periodontal disease. *Odontology.* 2004 Sep;92(1):1-8. doi: 10.1007/s10266-004-0043-4. PMID: 15490298.

[12] Kerdvongbundit V, Wikesjö UM. Effect of smoking on periodontal health in molar teeth. *J Periodontol.* 2000 Mar;71(3):433-7. doi: 10.1902/jop.2000.71.3.433. PMID: 10776931.

[13] Gera I. A dohányzás hatása a fogágybetegség elterjedtségére és gyakoriságára [The effect of smoking on the spread and frequency of periodontal disease].

Fogorv Sz. 1999 Apr;92(4):99–110. Hungarian. PMID: 10334078.

[14] Albandar JM, Streckfus CF, Adesanya MR, Winn DM. Cigar, pipe, and cigarette smoking as risk factors for periodontal disease and tooth loss. *J Periodontol.* 2000 Dec;71(12):1874–81. doi: 10.1902/jop.2000.71.12.1874. PMID:11156044.

[15] Bergström J, Eliasson S, Dock J. A 10- year prospective study of tobacco smoking and periodontal health. *J Periodontol.* 2000 Aug;71(8):1338–47. doi: 10.1902/ jop.2000.71.8.1338. PMID: 10972650.

[16] Johnson GK, Hill M. Cigarette smoking and the periodontal patient. *J Periodontol.* 2004 Feb;75(2):196–209. doi: 10.1902/ jop.2004.75.2.196. PMID: 15068107.

[17] Centers for Disease Control and Prevention. Highlights: smoking among adults in the United States: other health effects. [last updated 2015 Jul 15; cited 2018 Mar 22]. https://www.cdc.gov/tobacco/ data_statistics/sgr/2004/highlights/other_effects/ index.htm

[18] U.S. Department of Health and Human Services. A report of the Surgeon General. The health consequences of smoking. Atlanta: U.S. Department

of Health and Human Services, Centers for Disease Control and Prevention, National Center for Chronic Disease Prevention and Health Promotion, Office on Smoking and Health, 2004 [cited 2018 Mar 22]. PMID: 20669512.

[19] U.S. Department of Health and Human Services. The health consequences of smoking—50 years of progress: A report of the Surgeon General. Atlanta: U.S. Department of Health and Human Services, Centers for Disease Control and Prevention, National Center for Chronic Disease Prevention and Health Promotion, Office on Smoking and Health, 2014 [cited 2018 Mar 22]

[20] Eke PI, Dye BA, Wei L, et al. Prevalence of periodontitis in adults in the United States: 2009 and 2010. *J Dent Res.* 2012 Oct;91(10):914–20. doi: 10.1177002203 4512457373/. Epub 2012 Aug 30. PMID: 22935673. [cited 2018 Mar 22].

[21] U.S. Department of Health and Human Services. A report of the Surgeon General. The health consequences of smoking. Atlanta: U.S. Department of Health and Human Services, Centers for Disease Control and Prevention, National Center for Chronic Disease Prevention and Health Promotion, Office

on Smoking and Health, 2004 [cited 2018 Mar 22]. PMID: 20669512.

[22] National Institute of Dental and Craniofacial Research. Periodontal (gum) disease: causes, symptoms, and treatments. 2017. https://www.nidcr.nih.gov/sites/default/files/2017-09/ periodontal-disease_0.pdf [cited 2018 Mar 22].

[23] Hempton TJ, Leone C. The effects of smoking on periodontal disease and periodontal therapies. *J Mass Dent Soc.* 1997 Spring;46(1):33-5, 38-40. PMID: 9540728.

[24] Johnson GK, Guthmiller JM. The impact of cigarette smoking on periodontal disease and treatment. *Periodontol* 2000. 2007;44:178-94. doi: 10.1111/j.1600-0757.2007.00212.x. PMID: 17474933.

[25] Rota MT, Poggi P, Baratta L, Gaeta E, Boratto R, Tazzi A. Tobacco smoke in the development and therapy of periodontal disease: progress and questions. *Bull Group Int Rech Sci Stomatol Odontol.* 1999 Oct-Dec;41(4):116-22. doi: 10.3201/eid0801.010049. PMID: 11799741.

[26] Laxman VK, Annaji S. Tobacco use and its effects on the periodontium and periodontal therapy. *J Contemp Dent Pract.* 2008 Nov 1;9(7):97-107. PMID: 18997922.

[27] Centers for Disease Control and Prevention. Adult Oral Health: Facts About Adult Oral Health. Available from: https://www.cdc.gov/oralhealth/basics/adult-oral-health/index.html

[28] Silverstein P. Smoking and wound healing. *Am J Med.* 1992 Jul 15;93(1A):22S-24S. doi: 10.10160002/-9343(92)90623-j. PMID: 1323208.

[29] Netscher DT, Clamon J. Smoking: adverse effects on outcomes for plastic surgical patients. *Plast Surg Nurs.* 1994 Winter;14(4):205-10. doi: 10.109700006527/-199401440-00003. PMID: 7732100.

[30] Rinker B. The evils of nicotine: an evidence-based guide to smoking and plastic surgery. *Ann Plast Surg.* 2013 May;70(5):599-605. doi: 10.1097/SAP.0b013e3182764fcd. PMID: 23542839.

[31] Wright E, Tzeng TH, Ginnetti M, El-Othmani MM, Saleh JK, Saleh J, Lane JM, Mihalko WM, Saleh KJ. Effect of smoking on joint replacement outcomes: opportunities for improvement through preoperative smoking cessation. Instr Course Lect. 2016;65:509-20. PMID: 27049216.

[32] Whiteford L. Nicotine, CO and HCN: the detrimental effects of smoking on wound healing.

Br J Community Nurs. 2003 Dec;8(12):S22-6. doi: 10.12968/bjcn.2003.8.Sup6.12554. PMID: 14700008.

[33] Frick WG, Seals RR Jr. Smoking and wound healing: a review. *Tex Dent J.* 1994 Jun;111(6):21-3. PMID: 8633290.

[34] Marcy TW, Merrill WW. Cigarette smoking and respiratory tract infection. *Clin Chest Med.* 1987 Sep;8(3):381-91. PMID: 3311582.

[35] Ebihara S, Ebihara T, Okazaki T, Sasaki H. Cigarette smoking, cough reflex, and respiratory tract infection. *Arch Intern Med.* 2005 Apr 11;165(7):814. doi: 10.1001/archinte.165.7.814-a. PMID: 15824305.

[36] Marcy TW, Merrill WW. Cigarette smoking and respiratory tract infection. *Clin Chest Med.* 1987 Sep;8(3):381-91. PMID: 3311582.

[37] Peiffer G, Underner M, Perriot J. Les effets respiratoires du tabagisme [The respiratory effects of smoking]. *Rev Pneumol Clin.* 2018 Jun;74(3):133-144. French. doi: 10.1016/j. pneumo.2018.04.009. Epub 2018 May 22. PMID: 29793770.

[38] Ishii Y. Smoking and respiratory diseases. *Nihon Rinsho.* 2013 Mar;71(3):416-20. Japanese. PMID: 23631228.

[39] Milner D. The physiological effects of smoking on the respiratory system. *Nurs Times.* 2004 Jun 15-21;100(24):56-9. PMID: 15224495.

[40] McEvoy CT, Spindel ER. Pulmonary effects of maternal smoking on the fetus and child: effects on lung development, respiratory morbidities, and life-long lung health. *Paediatr Respir Rev.* 2017 Jan;21:27-33. doi: 10.1016/j. prrv.2016.08.005. Epub 2016 Aug 19. PMID: 27639458; PMCID: PMC5303131.

[41] Noël A, Hansen S, Zaman A, Perveen Z, Pinkston R, Hossain E, Xiao R, Penn A. In utero exposures to electronic-cigarette aerosols impair the *Wnt* signaling during mouse lung development. *Am J Physiol Lung Cell Mol Physiol.* 2020 Apr 1;318(4):L705-L722. doi: 10.1152/ajplung.00408.2019. Epub 2020 Feb 21. PMID: 32083945.

[41] Spindel ER, McEvoy CT. The role of nicotine in the effects of maternal smoking during pregnancy on lung development and childhood respiratory disease. Implications for dangers of E-cigarettes. *Am J Respir Crit Care Med.* 2016 Mar 1;193(5):486-94. doi: 10.1164/ rccm.201510-2013PP. PMID: 26756937; PMCID: PMC4824926.

[42] Lødrup Carlsen KC, Skjerven HO, Carlsen KH. The toxicity of E-cigarettes and children's respiratory health. *Paediatr Respir Rev.* 2018 Sep;28:63-67. doi: 10.1016/j.prrv.2018.01.002. Epub 2018 Feb 10. PMID: 29580719.

[43] Orzabal MR, Lunde-Young ER, Ramirez JI, Howe SYF, Naik VD, Lee J, Heaps CL,

[44] Threadgill DW, Ramadoss J. Chronic exposure to e-cig aerosols during early development causes vascular dysfunction and offspring growth deficits. *Transl Res.* 2019 May;207:70-82. doi: 10.1016/j. trsl.2019.01.001. Epub 2019 Jan 7. PMID: 30653941; PMCID: PMC6486852.

[45] Wong MK, Barra NG, Alfaidy N, Hardy DB, Holloway AC. Adverse effects of perinatal nicotine exposure on reproductive outcomes. *Reproduction.* 2015 Dec;150(6):R185-93. doi: 10.1530/REP-15-0295. Epub 2015 Oct 2. PMID: 26432348.

[46] Pereira PP, Da Mata FA, Figueiredo AC, de Andrade KR, Pereira MG. Maternal active smoking during pregnancy and low birth weight in the Americas: a systematic review and meta-analysis. *Nicotine Tob Res.* 2017 May 1;19(5):497-505. doi: 10.1093/ntr/ntw228. PMID: 28403455.

[47] Dessì A, Corona L, Pintus R, Fanos V. Exposure to tobacco smoke and low birth weight: from epidemiology to metabolomics. *Expert Rev Proteomics*. 2018 Aug;15(8):647–656. doi: 10.108014789450/.2018.1505508. Epub 2018 Aug 3. PMID: 30052087.

[48] Ko TJ, Tsai LY, Chu LC, Yeh SJ, Leung C, Chen CY, Chou HC, Tsao PN, Chen PC, Hsieh WS. Parental smoking during pregnancy and its association with low birth weight, small for gestational age, and preterm birth offspring: a birth cohort study. *Pediatr Neonatol*. 2014 Feb;55(1):20–7. doi: 10.1016/j. pedneo.2013.05.005. Epub 2013 Jul 12. PMID: 23850094.

[49] Wang R, Sun T, Yang Q, Yang Q, Wang J, Li H, Tang Y, Yang L, Sun J. Low birthweight of children is positively associated with mother's prenatal tobacco smoke exposure in Shanghai: a cross-sectional study. *BMC Pregnancy Childbirth*. 2020 Oct 8;20(1):603. doi: 10.1186/ s12884-020-03307-x. PMID: 33032551; PMCID: PMC7542738.

[50] Horta BL, Victora CG, Menezes AM, Halpern R, Barros FC. Low birthweight, preterm births and intrauterine growth retardation in relation to

maternal smoking. *Paediatr Perinat Epidemiol.* 1997 Apr;11(2):140-51. doi: 10.1046/j.1365-3016.1997.d01-17.x. PMID: 9131707.

[51] Centers for Disease Control and Prevention. Available from: https//www.cdc.gov/tobacco/quit

HABIT # 5: SLEEP.

[1] Besedovsky L, Lange T, Haack M. The sleep- immune crosstalk in health and disease. *Physiol Rev.* 2019 Jul 1;99(3):1325-1380. doi: 10.1152/ physrev.00010.2018. PMID: 30920354; PMCID: PMC6689741.

[2] Irwin MR. Why sleep is important for health: a psychoneuroimmunology perspective. *Annu Rev Psychol.* 2015 Jan 3;66:143-72. doi: 10.1146/annurev-psych-010213-115205. Epub 2014 Jul 21. PMID: 25061767; PMCID: PMC4961463.

[3] Majde JA, Krueger JM. Links between the innate immune system and sleep. *J Allergy Clin Immunol.* 2005 Dec;116(6):1188-98. doi: 10.1016/j.jaci.2005.08.005. Epub 2005 Sep 28. PMID: 16337444.

[4] Bryant PA, Trinder J, Curtis N. Sick and tired: does sleep have a vital role in the immune system? *Nat Rev Immunol.* 2004 Jun;4(6):457-67. doi: 10.1038/nri1369. PMID: 15173834.

[5] Gamaldo CE, Shaikh AK, McArthur JC. The sleep-immunity relationship. *Neurol Clin.* 2012 Nov;30(4):1313-43. doi: 10.1016/j. ncl.2012.08.007. PMID: 23099140

[6] Lorton D, Lubahn CL, Estus C, Millar BA, Carter JL, Wood CA, Bellinger DL. Bidirectional communication between the brain and the immune system: implications for physiological sleep and disorders with disrupted sleep. *Neuroimmunomodulation.* 2006;13(5-6):357-74. doi: 10.1159000104864/. Epub 2007 Aug 6. PMID: 17709958.

[7] Hui L, Hua F, Diandong H, Hong Y. Effects of sleep and sleep deprivation on immunoglobulins and complement in humans. *Brain Behav Immun.* 2007 Mar;21(3):308-10. doi: 10.1016/j.bbi.2006.09.005. Epub 2006 Oct 27. Erratum in: *Brain Behav Immun.* 2010 May;24(4).678-9. PMID. 17070668.

[8] Oztürk L, Pelin Z, Karadeniz D, Kaynak H, Cakar L, Gözükirmizi E. Effects of 48 hours sleep deprivation on human immune profile. *Sleep Res Online.* 1999;2(4):107-11. PMID: 11382891.

[9] Rogers NL, Szuba MP, Staab JP, Evans DL, Dinges DF. Neuroimmunologic aspects of sleep and sleep loss.

Semin Clin Neuropsychiatry. 2001 Oct;6(4):295-307. doi: 10.1053/ scnp.2001.27907. PMID: 11607924.

[10] Wilder-Smith A, Mustafa FB, Earnest A, Gen L, Macary PA. Impact of partial sleep deprivation on immune markers. *Sleep Med.* 2013 Oct;14(10):1031-4. doi: 10.1016/j.sleep.2013.07.001. Epub 2013 Aug 28. PMID:23993876.

[11] Nami M, Mehrabi S, Kamali AM, Kazemiha M, Carvalho J, Derman S, Lakey-Betia J, Vasquez V, Kosagisharaf R. A new hypothesis on anxiety, sleep insufficiency, and viral infections; reciprocal links to consider in today's "World vs. COVID-19". Endeavors. *Front Psychiatry.* 2020 Nov 5;11:585893. doi: 10.3389/fpsyt.2020.585893. PMID: 33250794; PMCID: PMC7674554.

[12] Besedovsky L, Lange T, Born J. Sleep and immune function. *Pflugers Arch.* 2012 Jan;463(1):121-37. doi: 10.1007/s00424-011- 1044-0. Epub 2011 Nov 10. PMID: 22071480; PMCID: PMC3256323.

[13] Lange T, Dimitrov S, Bollinger T, Diekelmann S, Born J. Sleep after vaccination boosts immunological memory. *J Immunol.* 2011 Jul 1;187(1):283-90. doi: 10.4049/jimmunol.1100015. Epub 2011 Jun 1. PMID: 21632713.

[14] Silva ESME, Ono BHVS, Souza JC. Sleep and immunity in times of COVID-19. *Rev Assoc Med Bras* (1992). 2020 Sep 21;66Suppl 2(Suppl 2):143-147. doi: 10.15901806/-9282.66.S2.143. PMID: 32965373.

[15] Prather AA, Janicki-Deverts D, Hall MH, Cohen S. Behaviorally assessed sleep and susceptibility to the common cold. *Sleep.* 2015 Sep 1;38(9):1353-9. doi: 10.5665/sleep.4968. PMID: 26118561; PMCID: PMC4531403.

[16] Cohen S, Doyle WJ, Alper CM, Janicki- Deverts D, Turner RB. Sleep habits and susceptibility to the common cold. *Arch Intern Med.* 2009 Jan 12;169(1):62-7. doi: 10.1001/archinternmed.2008.505. PMID: 19139325; PMCID: PMC2629403.

[17] Spiegel K, Sheridan JF, Van Cauter E. Effect of sleep deprivation on response to immunization. *JAMA* 2002;288(12):1471-1472.

[18] Irwin MR, Mascovich A, Gillin JC, Willoughby R, Pike J, Smith TL [1994]. Partial sleep deprivation reduces natural killer cell activity in humans. *Psychosom Med*;56(6):493-498.

[19] U.S. Department of Health and Human Services. Office of Disease Prevention and Health Promotion. *Healthy people* 2020 sleep health. Available from: http://www.healthypeople.gov/2020/topics-objectives/topic/sleep-healthexternal icon

[20] National Heart, Lung, and Blood Institute, National Institutes of Health. How much sleep is enough? 2012. Available from: http://www.nhlbi.nih.gov/health/health-topics/topics/sdd/howmuchexternal icon

[21] Sleep.org. How is sleep quantity different from sleep quality. Available from: https://www.sleep.org/sleep-quantity-different-sleep-quality/#:~:text=Unlike%20sleep%20quantity%2C%20sleep%20quality,if%20you%20do%20wake%20up.

[22] National Heart, Lung, and Blood Institute, National Institutes of Health. How much sleep is enough? 2012. Available from: http://www.nhlbi.nih.gov/health/health-topics/topics/sdd/howmuchexternal icon

[23] Luckhaupt SE, Tak SW, Calvert GM [2010]. The prevalence of short sleep duration by industry and occupation in the National Health Interview Survey. *Sleep*;33:149-159.

[24] Liu Y, Wheaton AG, Chapman DP, Croft JB. Sleep duration and chronic diseases among US

adults age 45 years and older: evidence from the 2010 Behavioral Risk Factor Surveillance System. *Sleep* 2013;36(10):1421-1427.

[25] Caldwell JA, Mallis MM, Caldwell JL, Paul MA, Miller JC, Neri DF, Aerospace Medical Association Fatigue Countermeasures Subcommittee of the Aerospace Human Factors Committee. Fatigue countermeasures in aviation. *Aviation Space Environ Med* 2009;80(1):29–

[26] Sanassi LA. Seasonal affective disorder: is there light at the end of the tunnel? *JAAPA*. 2014 Feb;27(2):18–22;quiz 23. doi: 10.109701/. JAA.0000442698.03223. f3. PMID: 24394440.

[27] Tuunainen A, Kripke DF, Endo T. Light therapy for non–seasonal depression. *Cochrane Database Syst Rev.* 2004;2004(2):CD004050. doi: 10.100211651858/.CD004050.pub2. PMID: 15106233; PMCID: PMC6669243.

[28] Viola AU, James LM, Schlangen LJ, Dijk DJ. Blue-enriched white light in the workplace improves self–reported alertness, performance and sleep quality. *Scand J Work Environ Health.* 2008 Aug;34(4):297–306. doi: 10.5271/sjweh.1268. Epub 2008 Sep 22. PMID: 18815716.

[29] Fetveit A, Skjerve A, Bjorvatn B. Bright light treatment improves sleep in institutionalised elderly--an open trial. *Int J Geriatr Psychiatry.* 2003 Jun;18(6):520-6. doi: 10.1002/gps.852. PMID: 12789673.

[30] Fonken LK, Workman JL, Walton JC, Weil ZM, Morris JS, Haim A, Nelson RJ. Light at night increases body mass by shifting the time of food intake. *Proc Natl Acad Sci USA.* 2010 Oct 26;107(43):18664-9. doi: 10.1073/pnas.1008734107. Epub 2010 Oct 11. PMID: 20937863; PMCID: PMC2972983.

[31] Higuchi S, Motohashi Y, Liu Y, Maeda A. Effects of playing a computer game using a bright display on presleep physiological variables, sleep latency, slow wave sleep and REM sleep. *J Sleep Res.* 2005 Sep;14(3):267-73. doi: 10.1111/j.1365-2869.2005.00463.x. PMID: 16120101.

[32] Gooley, JJ, Chamberlain, K, Smith, KA, Khalsa, SB, Rajaratnam, SM, Van Reen, E, Zeitzer, JM, Czeisler, CA, & Lockley, SW. Exposure to room light before bedtime suppresses melatonin onset and shortens melatonin duration in humans. *The Journal of clinical*

endocrinology and metabolism. 2011;96(3), E463–E472. Available from: https://doi.org/10.1210/jc.2010-2098

[33] Figueiro MG, Wood B, Plitnick B, Rea MS. The impact of light from computer monitors on melatonin levels in college students. *Neuro Endocrinol Lett.* 2011;32(2):158-63. PMID: 21552190.

[34] Sasseville A, Paquet N, Sévigny J, Hébert M. Blue blocker glasses impede the capacity of bright light to suppress melatonin production. *J Pineal Res.* 2006 Aug;41(1):73-8. doi: 10.1111/j.1600-079X.2006.00332.x. PMID: 16842544.

[35] Groeger JA, Lo JC, Burns CG, Dijk DJ. Effects of sleep inertia after daytime naps vary with executive load and time of day. *Behav Neurosci.* 2011 Apr;125(2):252-60. doi: 10.1037/ a0022692. PMID: 21463024.

[36] McDevitt EA, Alaynick WA, Mednick SC. The effect of nap frequency on daytime sleep architecture. *Physiol Behav.* 2012 Aug 20;107(1):40-4. doi: 10.1016/j.physbeh.2012.05.021. Epub 2012 May 31. PMID: 22659474; PMCID: PMC3744392.

[37] Dhand R, Sohal H. Good sleep, bad sleep! The role of daytime naps in healthy adults. *Curr Opin*

Pulm Med. 2006 Nov;12(6):379-82. doi: 10.109701/.
mcp.0000245703.92311.d0. PMID: 17053484.

[38] Pilcher JJ, Michalowski KR, Carrigan RD. The
prevalence of daytime napping and its relationship to
nighttime sleep. *Behav Med.* 2001 Summer;27(2):71-6.
doi: 10.1080089642801109595773/. PMID: 11763827.

[39] Dautovich ND, McCrae CS, Rowe M. Subjective
and objective napping and sleep in older adults: are
evening naps "bad" for nighttime sleep? *J Am Geriatr
Soc.* 2008 Sep;56(9):1681-6. doi: 10.1111/j.1532-
5415.2008.01822.x. Epub 2008 Aug 5. PMID:
18691289; PMCID: PMC4020142.

[40] Van Dongen HP, Dinges DF. Investigating the
interaction between the homeostatic and circadian
processes of sleep-wake regulation for the prediction
of waking neurobehavioural performance. *J Sleep
Res.* 2003 Sep;12(3):181-7. doi: 10.1046/j.1365-
2869.2003.00357.x. PMID: 12941057.

[41] Giannotti F, Cortesi F, Sebastiani T, Ottaviano S.
Circadian preference, sleep and daytime behaviour
in adolescence. *J Sleep Res.* 2002 Sep;11(3):191-9. doi:
10.1046/j.1365-2869.2002.00302.x. PMID: 12220314.

[42] Baehr EK, Revelle W, Eastman CI. Individual
differences in the phase and amplitude of the

human circadian temperature rhythm: with an emphasis on morningness-eveningness. *J Sleep Res.* 2000 Jun;9(2):117-27. doi: 10.1046/j.1365-2869.2000.00196.x. PMID: 10849238.

[43] Emens JS, Yuhas K, Rough J, Kochar N, Peters D, Lewy AJ. Phase angle of entrainment in morning- and evening-types under naturalistic conditions. *Chronobiol Int.* 2009;26(3):474-493. doi:10.1080074205209028210 77/

[44] Issa FG, Sullivan CE. Alcohol, snoring and sleep apnea. *J Neurol Neurosurg Psychiatry.* 1982 Apr;45(4):353-9. doi: 10.1136/ jnnp.45.4.353. PMID: 7077345; PMCID: PMC491372.

[45] Taasan VC, Block AJ, Boysen PG, Wynne JW. Alcohol increases sleep apnea and oxygen desaturation in asymptomatic men. *Am J Med.* 1981 Aug;71(2).240-5. doi: 10.1016 0002-9343(81)90124-8. PMID: 7258218.

[46] Ekman AC, Leppäluoto J, Huttunen P, Aranko K, Vakkuri O. Ethanol inhibits melatonin secretion in healthy volunteers in a dose-dependent randomized double blind cross-over study. *J Clin Endocrinol Metab.* 1993 Sep;77(3):780-3. doi: 10.1210/jcem.77.3.8370699. PMID: 8370699.

[47] Stevens RG, Davis S, Mirick DK, Kheifets L, Kaune W. Alcohol consumption and urinary concentration of 6-sulfatoxymelatonin in healthy women. *Epidemiology*. 2000 Nov;11(6):660-5. doi: 10.109700001648/-200011000-00008. PMID: 11055626.

[48] Wetterberg, L., Aperia, B., Gorelick, D. A., Gwirtzman, H. E., McGuire, M. T., Serafetinides, E. A., & Yuwiler, A. Age, alcoholism and depression are associated with low levels of urinary melatonin. *Journal of psychiatry & neuroscience*. 1992;17(5), 215-224.

[49] Ekman AC, Vakkuri O, Ekman M, Leppäluoto J, Ruokonen A, Knip M. Ethanol decreases nocturnal plasma levels of thyrotropin and growth hormone but not those of thyroid hormones or prolactin in man. *J Clin Endocrinol Metab*. 1996 Jul;81(7):2627-32. doi: 10.1210/ jcem.81.7.8675588. PMID: 8675588.

[50] Libert JP, Bach V, Johnson LC, Ehrhart J, Wittersheim G, Keller D. Relative and combined effects of heat and noise exposure on sleep in humans. *Sleep*. 1991 Feb;14(1):24-31. doi: 10.1093/sleep/14.1.24. PMID: 1811316.

[51] Waye KP, Clow A, Edwards S, Hucklebridge F, Rylander R. Effects of nighttime low frequency noise on the cortisol response to awakening and subjective

sleep quality. *Life Sci.* 2003 Jan 10;72(8):863-75. doi: 10.1016/s0024- 3205(02)02336-6. PMID: 12493567.

[52] Halperin D. Environmental noise and sleep disturbances: a threat to health? *Sleep Sci.* 2014 Dec;7(4):209-12. doi: 10.1016/j.slsci.2014.11.003. Epub 2014 Nov 15. PMID: 26483931; PMCID: PMC4608916.

[53] Lee KA, Gay CL. Can modifications to the bedroom environment improve the sleep of new parents? Two randomized controlled trials. *Res Nurs Health.* 2011 Feb;34(1):7-19. doi: 10.1002/nur.20413. Epub 2010 Nov 17. PMID: 21243655; PMCID: PMC3066036.

[54] Okamoto-Mizuno K, Tsuzuki K, Mizuno K. Effects of mild heat exposure on sleep stages and body temperature in older men. *Int J Biometeorol.* 2004 Sep;49(1):32-6. doi: 10.1007/ s00484-004-0209-3. Epub 2004 Jun 2. PMID. 15173935.

[55] Libert JP, Di Nisi J, Fukuda H, Muzet A, Ehrhart J, Amoros C. Effect of continuous heat exposure on sleep stages in humans. *Sleep.* 1988 Apr;11(2):195-209. doi: 10.1093/sleep/11.2.195. PMID: 3381060.

[56] Okamoto-Mizuno K, Tsuzuki K, Mizuno K. Effects of humid heat exposure in later sleep segments on sleep stages and body temperature in

humans. *Int J Biometeorol.* 2005 Mar;49(4):232-7. doi: 10.1007/s00484-004- 0237-z. Epub 2004 Dec 1. PMID: 15578234.

[57] Di Nisi J, Ehrhart J, Galeou M, Libert JP. Influence of repeated passive body heating on subsequent night sleep in humans. *Eur J Appl Physiol Occup Physiol.* 1989;59(1-2):138-45. doi: 10.1007/BF02396592. PMID: 2583142.

[58] Lack LC, Gradisar M, Van Someren EJ, Wright HR, Lushington K. The relationship between insomnia and body temperatures. *Sleep Med Rev.* 2008 Aug;12(4):307-17. doi: 10.1016/j. smrv.2008.02.003. PMID: 18603220.

[59] Jalilolghadr S, Afaghi A, O'Connor H, Chow CM. Effect of low and high glycaemic index drink on sleep pattern in children. *J Pak Med Assoc.* 2011 Jun;61(6):533-6. PMID: 22204204.

[60] Allison KC, Lundgren JD, O'Reardon JP, Geliebter A, Gluck ME, Vinai P, Mitchell JE, Schenck CH, Howell MJ, Crow SJ, Engel S, Latzer Y, Tzischinsky O, Mahowald MW, Stunkard AJ. Proposed diagnostic criteria for night eating syndrome. *Int J Eat Disord.* 2010 Apr;43(3):241-7. doi: 10.1002/eat.20693. PMID: 19378289; PMCID: PMC4531092.

[61] Schenck CH, Mahowald MW. Review of nocturnal sleep-related eating disorders. *Int J Eat Disord*. 1994 May;15(4):343-56. doi: 10.1002/eat.2260150405. PMID: 8032349.

[62] Howell MJ, Schenck CH, Crow SJ. A review of nighttime eating disorders. *Sleep Med Rev*. 2009 Feb;13(1):23-34. doi: 10.1016/j. smrv.2008.07.005. Epub 2008 Sep 25. PMID: 18819825.

[63] Vander Wal JS. Night eating syndrome: a critical review of the literature. *Clin Psychol Rev*. 2012 Feb;32(1):49-59. doi: 10.1016/j.cpr.2011.11.001. Epub 2011 Nov 9. PMID: 22142838.

[64] Liao WC, Landis CA, Lentz MJ, Chiu MJ. Effect of foot bathing on distal-proximal skin temperature gradient in elders. *Int J Nurs Stud*. 2005 Sep;42(7):717-22. doi: 10.1016/j.ijnurstu.2004.11.011. Epub 2005 Jan 25. PMID: 16084919.

[65] Kanda K, Tochihara Y, Ohnaka T. Bathing before sleep in the young and in the elderly. *Eur J Appl Physiol Occup Physiol*. 1999 Jul;80(2):71-5. doi: 10.1007/s004210050560. PMID: 10408315.

[66] Liao WC. Effects of passive body heating on body temperature and sleep regulation in the elderly: a systematic review. *Int J Nurs Stud*. 2002

Nov;39(8):803-10. doi: 10.1016/s0020-7489(02)00023-8. PMID: 12379298.

[67] Liao WC, Chiu MJ, Landis CA. A warm footbath before bedtime and sleep in older Taiwanese with sleep disturbance. *Res Nurs Health.* 2008 Oct;31(5):514-28. doi: 10.1002/nur.20283. PMID: 18459154; PMCID: PMC2574895.

[68] Sung EJ, Tochihara Y. Effects of bathing and hot footbath on sleep in winter. *J Physiol Anthropol Appl Human Sci.* 2000 Jan;19(1):21-7. doi: 10.2114/jpa.19.21. PMID: 10979246.

[69] Coursey RD, Frankel BL, Gaarder KR, Mott DE. A comparison of relaxation techniques with electrosleep therapy for chronic, sleep-onset insomnia a sleep-EEG study. *Biofeedback Self Regul.* 1980 Mar;5(1):57-73. doi: 10.1007/ BF00999064. PMID: 6989409.

[70] Friedman L, Bliwise DL, Yesavage JA, Salom SR. A preliminary study comparing sleep restriction and relaxation treatments for insomnia in older adults. *J Gerontol.* 1991 Jan;46(1):P1-8. doi: 10.1093/ geronj/46.1.p1. PMID: 1986039.

[71] Rider MS, Floyd JW, Kirkpatrick J. The effect of music, therapy, and relaxation on adrenal corticosteroids and the re-entrainment of circadian

rhythms. *J Music Ther.* 1985 Spring;22(1):46-58. doi: 10.1093/jmt/22.1.46. PMID: 10271532.

[72] Richards KC. Effect of a back massage and relaxation intervention on sleep in critically ill patients. *Am J Crit Care.* 1998 Jul;7(4):288-99. PMID: 9656043.

[73] Phillipson EA. Sleep apnea--a major public health problem. *N Engl J Med.* 1993 Apr 29;328(17):1271-3. doi: 10.1056/ NEJM199304293281712. PMID: 8464440.

[74] Young T, Skatrud J, Peppard PE. Risk factors for obstructive sleep apnea in adults. *JAMA.* 2004 Apr 28;291(16):2013-6. doi: 10.1001/jama.291.16.2013. PMID: 15113821.

[75] Young T, Palta M, Dempsey J, Skatrud J, Weber S, Badr S. The occurrence of sleep-disordered breathing among middle-aged adults. *N Engl J Med.* 1993 Apr 29;328(17):1230-5. doi: 10.1056/ NEJM199304293281704. PMID: 8464434.

[76] Aurora, RN, et al. The treatment of restless legs syndrome and periodic limb movement disorder in adults--an update for 2012: practice parameters with an evidence-based systematic review and meta-analyses: an American Academy of Sleep Medicine

Clinical Practice Guideline. *Sleep* 2012 Aug 1;35,8 1039-62. doi:10.5665/sleep.1988

[77] Zhu, L, and Zee, PC. Circadian rhythm sleep disorders. *Neurologic clinics* 2012;30(4): 1167-91. doi:10.1016/j.ncl.2012.08.011

[78] Jacobson BH, Boolani A, Dunklee G, Shepardson A, Acharya H. Effect of prescribed sleep surfaces on back pain and sleep quality in patients diagnosed with low back and shoulder pain. Appl Ergon. 2010 Dec;42(1):91-7. doi: 10.1016/j.apergo.2010.05.004. Epub 2010 Jun 26. PMID: 20579971.

[79] Marin R, Cyhan T, Miklos W. Sleep disturbance in patients with chronic low back pain. *Am J Phys Med Rehabil.* 2006 May;85(5):430-5. doi: 10.109701/. phm.0000214259.06380.79. PMID: 16628150.

[80] Jacobson BH, Gemmell HA, Hayes BM, Altena TS. Effectiveness of a selected bedding system on quality of sleep, low back pain, shoulder pain, and spine stiffness. *J Manipulative Physiol Ther.* 2002 Feb;25(2):88-92. doi: 10.1067/ mmt.2002.121410. PMID: 11896375.

[81] Jacobson, BH, et al. Changes in back pain, sleep quality, and perceived stress after introduction of new bedding systems. *Journal of chiropractic medicine* 2009;8(1):1-8. doi:10.1016/j.jcm.2008.09.002

[82] Bader GG, Engdal S. The influence of bed firmness on sleep quality. *Appl Ergon.* 2000 Oct;31(5):487-97. doi: 10.1016/s0003- 6870(00)00013-2. PMID: 11059462.

[83] Jacobson BH, Wallace TJ, Smith DB, Kolb T. Grouped comparisons of sleep quality for new and personal bedding systems. *Appl Ergon.* 2008 Mar;39(2):247-54. doi: 10.1016/j. apergo.2007.04.002. Epub 2007 Jun 26. PMID: 17597575.

[84] Reid KJ, Baron KG, Lu B, Naylor E, Wolfe L, Zee PC. Aerobic exercise improves self-reported sleep and quality of life in older adults with insomnia. *Sleep Med.* 2010 Oct;11(9):934-40. doi: 10.1016/j. sleep.2010.04.014. Epub 2010 Sep 1. PMID: 20813580; PMCID: PMC2992829.

[85] Yang PY, Ho KH, Chen HC, Chien MY. Exercise training improves sleep quality in middle-aged and older adults with sleep problems: a systematic review. *J Physiother.* 2012;58(3):157-63. doi: 10.1016/S1836- 9553(12)70106-6. PMID: 22884182.

[86] Youngstedt SD. Effects of exercise on sleep. *Clin Sports Med.* 2005 Apr;24(2):355-65, xi. doi: 10.1016/j. csm.2004.12.003. PMID: 15892929.

[87] King AC, Oman RF, Brassington GS, Bliwise DL, Haskell WL. Moderate-intensity exercise and self-rated quality of sleep in older adults. A randomized controlled trial. *JAMA*. 1997 Jan 1;277(1):32-7. PMID: 8980207.

[88] Lira FS, Pimentel GD, Santos RV, Oyama LM, Damaso AR, Oller do Nascimento CM, Viana VA, Boscolo RA, Grassmann V, Santana MG, Esteves AM, Tufik S, de Mello MT. Exercise training improves sleep pattern and metabolic profile in elderly people in a time-dependent manner. *Lipids Health Dis*. 2011 Jul 6;10:1-6. doi: 10.11861476/-511X-10-113. PMID: 21733182; PMCID: PMC3154859.

[89] Passos GS, Poyares D, Santana MG, Garbuio SA, Tufik S, Mello MT. Effect of acute physical exercise on patients with chronic primary insomnia. *J Clin Sleep Med*. 2010 Jun 15;6(3):270-5. PMID: 20572421; PMCID: PMC2883039.

[90] Marschall-Kehrel D. Update on nocturia: the best of rest is sleep. *Urology*. 2004 Dec;64(6 Suppl 1):21-4. doi: 10.1016/j. urology.2004.10.072. PMID: 15621224.

[91] Asplund R. Nocturia, nocturnal polyuria, and sleep quality in the elderly. *J Psychosom*

Res. 2004 May;56(5):517-25. doi: 10.1016/j. jpsychores.2004.04.003. PMID: 15172208.

HABIT # 6: Get Your Ex Back!

[1] Nieman DC, Wentz LM. The compelling link between physical activity and the body's defense system. *J Sport Health Sci.* 2019 May;8(3):201-217. doi: 10.1016/j.jshs.2018.09.009. Epub 2018 Nov 16. PMID: 31193280; PMCID: PMC6523821.

[2] Idorn M, Thor Straten P. Exercise and cancer: from "healthy" to "therapeutic"? *Cancer Immunol Immunother.* 2017 May;66(5):667-671. doi: 10.1007/ s00262-017-1985-z. Epub 2017 Mar 21. PMID: 28324125; PMCID: PMC5406418.

[3] Ashcraft KA, Warner AB, Jones LW, Dewhirst MW. Exercise as adjunct therapy in cancer. *Semin Radiat Oncol.* 2019 Jan;29(1):16-24. doi: 10.1016/j. semradonc.2018.10.001. PMID: 30573180; PMCID: PMC6656408.

[4] Tschentscher M, Niederseer D, Niebauer J. Health benefits of Nordic walking: a systematic review. *Am J Prev Med.* 2013 Jan;44(1):76-84. doi: 10.1016/j. amepre.2012.09.043. PMID: 23253654.

[5] Simpson RJ, Kunz H, Agha N, Graff R. Exercise and the regulation of immune functions. *Prog Mol Biol Transl Sci.* 2015;135:355-80. doi: 10.1016/bs.pmbts.2015.08.001. Epub 2015 Sep 5. PMID: 26477922

[6] Simpson RJ, Campbell JP, Gleeson M, Krüger K, Nieman DC, Pyne DB, Turner JE, Walsh NP. Can exercise affect immune function to increase susceptibility to infection? *Exerc Immunol Rev.* 2020;26:8-22. PMID: 32139352.

[7] Trochimiak T, Hübner-Woźniak E. Effect of exercise on the level of immunoglobulin a in saliva. *Biol Sport.* 2012 Dec;29(4):255-61. doi: 10.560420831862/.1019662. Epub 2012 Nov PMID: 24868115; PMCID: PMC4033058.

[8] da Silveira MP, da Silva Fagundes KK, Bizuti MR, Starck É, Rossi RC, de Resende E Silva DT. Physical exercise as a tool to help the immune system against COVID-19: an integrative review of the current literature. *Clin Exp Med.* 2020 Jul 29:1–14. doi: 10.1007/s10238-020-00650-3. Epub ahead of print. PMID: 32728975; PMCID: PMC7387807.

[9] Yang PY, Ho KH, Chen HC, Chien MY. Exercise training improves sleep quality in middle-aged and

older adults with sleep problems: a systematic review. *J Physiother.* 2012;58(3):157-63. doi: 10.1016/S1836-9553(12)70106-6. PMID: 22884182.

[10] King AC, Oman RF, Brassington GS, Bliwise DL, Haskell WL. Moderate-intensity exercise and self-rated quality of sleep in older adults. A randomized controlled trial. *JAMA* 1997 Jan 1;277(1):32-7. PMID: 8980207.

[11] Reid KJ, Baron KG, Lu B, Naylor E, Wolfe L, Zee PC. Aerobic exercise improves self-reported sleep and quality of life in older adults with insomnia. *Sleep Med.* 2010 Oct;11(9):934-40. doi: 10.1016/j. sleep.2010.04.014. Epub 2010 Sep 1. PMID: 20813580; PMCID: PMC2992829.

[12] Passos GS, Poyares D, Santana MG, D'Aurea CV, Youngstedt SD, Tufik S, de Mello MT. Effects of moderate aerobic exercise training on chronic primary insomnia. *Sleep Med.* 2011 Dec;12(10):1018-27. doi: 10.1016/j. sleep.2011.02.007. Epub 2011 Oct 22. PMID: 22019457.

[13] Amanat S, Ghahri S, Dianatinasab A, Fararouei M, Dianatinasab M. Exercise and Type 2 Diabetes. *Adv Exp Med Biol.* 2020;1228:91-105. doi: 10.1007978/-981-15-1792-1_6. PMID: 32342452.

[14] Wallberg-Henriksson H, Rincon J, Zierath JR. Exercise in the management of non-insulin-dependent diabetes mellitus. *Sports Med.* 1998 Jan;25(1):25-35. doi: 10.216500007256/-199825010-00003. Erratum in: Sports Med 1998 Feb;25(2):130. PMID: 9458525.

[15] Lehmann R, Spinas GA. Die Rolle der körperlichen Aktivität in der Therapie und für die Prävention des Typ-II-Diabetes mellitus [Role of physical activity in the therapy and prevention of Type II diabetes mellitus]. *Ther Umsch.* 1996 Dec;53(12):925-33. German. PMID: 9036570.

[16] Ivy JL. Role of exercise training in the prevention and treatment of insulin resistance and non-insulin-dependent diabetes mellitus. *Sports Med.* 1997 Nov;24(5):321-36. doi: 10.216500007256/-199724050-00004. PMID: 9368278.

[17] Pedersen BK, Saltin B. Evidence for prescribing exercise as therapy in chronic disease. *Scand J Med Sci Sports.* 2006 Feb;16 Suppl 1:3-63. doi: 10.1111/j.1600-0838.2006.00520.x. PMID: 16451303.

[18] Moraes-Silva IC, Mostarda CT, Silva-Filho AC, Irigoyen MC. Hypertension and exercise training: evidence from clinical studies. *Adv Exp Med Biol.*

2017;1000:65-84. doi: 10.1007978/- 981-10-4304-8_5.
PMID: 29098616.

[19] Pedersen BK, Saltin B. Exercise as medicine -
evidence for prescribing exercise as therapy in 26
different chronic diseases. *Scand J Med Sci Sports.*
2015 Dec;25 Suppl 3:1-72. doi: 10.1111/ sms.12581.
PMID: 26606383.

[20] Arija V, Villalobos F, Pedret R, Vinuesa A, Jovani D,
Pascual G, Basora J. Physical activity, cardiovascular
health, quality of life and blood pressure control
in hypertensive subjects: randomized clinical trial.
Health Qual Life Outcomes. 2018 Sep 14;16(1):184.
doi: 10.1186/s12955-018-1008-6. PMID: 30217193;
PMCID: PMC6137925.

[21] Toups M, Carmody T, Greer T, Rethorst C,
Grannemann B, Trivedi MH. Exercise is an effective
treatment for positive valence symptoms in major
depression. *J Affect Disord.* 2017 Feb;209:188-194. doi:
10.1016/j. jad.2016.08.058. Epub 2016 Oct 15. PMID:
27936452; PMCID: PMC6036912.

[22] Callaghan P. Exercise: a neglected intervention
in mental health care? *J Psychiatr Ment Health
Nurs.* 2004 Aug;11(4):476-83. doi: 10.1111/j.1365-
2850.2004.00751.x. PMID: 15255923.

[23] Lubans D, Richards J, Hillman C, Faulkner G, Beauchamp M, Nilsson M, Kelly P, Smith J, Raine L, Biddle S. Physical activity for cognitive and mental health in youth: a systematic review of mechanisms. *Pediatrics.* 2016 Sep;138(3):e20161642. doi: 10.1542/peds.2016-1642. Epub 2016 Aug 19. PMID: 27542849.

[24] Biddle SJ, Asare M. Physical activity and mental health in children and adolescents: a review of reviews. *Br J Sports Med.* 2011 Sep;45(11):886-95. doi: 10.1136/bjsports-2011-090185. Epub 2011 Aug 1. PMID: 21807669.

[25] Mikkelsen K, Stojanovska L, Polenakovic M, Bosevski M, Apostolopoulos V. Exercise and mental health. *Maturitas.* 2017 Dec;106:48-56. doi: 10.1016/j.maturitas.2017.09.003. Epub 2017 Sep 7. PMID: 29150166.

[26] Puterman E, Weiss J, Lin J, Schilf S, Slusher AL, Johansen KL, Epel ES. Aerobic exercise lengthens telomeres and reduces stress in family caregivers: a randomized controlled trial - Curt Richter Award Paper 2018. *Psychoneuroendocrinology.* 2018 Dec;98:245-252. doi: 10.1016/j.psyneuen.2018.08.002. Epub 2018 Aug 2. PMID: 30266522.

[27] What are the different types of walking – Walking Academy Available from: https://walkingacademy.com/what-are-the-different-types-of-walking

HABIT # 7: LAUGH

[1] Bennett MP, Zeller JM, Rosenberg L, McCann J. The effect of mirthful laughter on stress and natural killer cell activity. *Altern Ther Health Med.* 2003;9(2):38-45.

[2] Takahashi K, Iwase M, Yamashita K, et al. The elevation of natural killer cell activity induced by laughter in a crossover-designed study. *Int J Molecular Med.* 2001;8(6);645-650.

[3] McClelland R, Cheriff A. The immunoenhancing effects of humour on secretory IgA and resistance to respiratory infections. *Psychol Health.*1997;12(3):329-344.

[4] Lefcourt H, Davidson-Katz K, Kueneman K. Humor and immune system functioning. *Humor: Int J Humor Res.* 1990;3:305-321.

[5] Dillon KM, Minchoff B, Baker KH. Positive emotional status and enhancement of the immune system. *Int J Psychiatry Med.* 1985- 1986;15(1):13-18.

[6] Labott SM, Ahleman S, Wolever ME, Martin RB. The physiological and psychological effects

of the expression and inhibition of emotion. *Behav Med.* 1990;16(4):182-189.

[7] Martin RA, Dobbin JP. Sense of humor, hassles, and immunoglobulin A: evidence for a stress- moderating effect of humor. *Int J Psychiatry Med.* 1988;18(2):93105.

[8] Kimata H. Reduction of plasma levels of neurotrophins by laughter in patients with atopic dermatitis. *Pediatr Asthma Allergy Immunol.* 2004;17(2):131-135.

[9] Dunbar RI, Baron R, Frangou A, Pearce E, van Leeuwen EJ, Stow J, Partridge G, MacDonald I, Barra V, van Vugt M. Social laughter is correlated with an elevated pain threshold. *Proc Biol Sci.* 2012 Mar 22;279(1731):1161-7. doi: 10.1098/ rspb.2011.1373. Epub 2011 Sep 14. PMID: 21920973; PMCID: PMC3267132.

[10] Stuber M, Hilber SD, Mintzer LL, Castaneda M, Glover D, Zeltzer L. Laughter, humor and pain perception in children: a pilot study. *Evid Based Complement Alternat Med.* 2009 Jun;6(2):271-6. doi: 10.1093/ecam/nem097. Epub 2007 Oct 5. PMID: 18955244; PMCID: PMC2686629.

[11] Lapierre SS, Baker BD, Tanaka H. Effects of mirthful laughter on pain tolerance: a randomized controlled

investigation. *J Bodyw Mov Ther.* 2019 Oct;23(4):733-738. doi: 10.1016/j.jbmt.2019.04.005. Epub 2019 Apr 13. PMID: 31733755.

[12] Pérez-Aranda A, Hofmann J, Feliu-Soler A, Ramírez-Maestre C, Andrés-Rodríguez L, Ruch W, Luciano JV. Laughing away the pain: a narrative review of humour, sense of humour and pain. *Eur J Pain.* 2019 Feb;23(2):220-233. doi: 10.1002/ejp.1309. Epub 2018 Sep 30. PMID: 30176100.

[13] Fight stress with healthy habits infographic. American Heart Association. Available from: https://www.heart.org/en/healthy-living/healthy-lifestyle/stress-management/fight-stress-with-healthy-habits-infographic#.VtB5i9j2bIU. Cited March 11, 2019.

[14] Woodbury-Farina MA, et al. Humor. *Psychiatric Clinics of North America.* 2014;37:561.

[15] Wilkins J, et al. Humor theories and the physiological benefits of laughter. *Holistic Nursing Practice.* 2009;23:349.

[16] Sridharan K, et al. Therapeutic clowns in pediatrics: a systematic review and meta- analysis of randomized controlled trials. *European Journal of Pediatrics.* 2016;175:1353.

[17] Savage BM, et al. Humor, laughter, learning, and health! A brief review. *Advances in Physiology Education*. 2017;41:341.

[18] Chang C, et al. Psychological, immunological and physiological effects of a Laughing Qigong Program (LQP) on adolescents. *Complementary Therapies in Medicine*. 2013;21:660.

[19] Seaward BL. Comic relief: The healing power of humor. In: Essentials of Managing Stress. 4th ed. Burlington, Mass.: Jones & Bartlett Learning 2017.

[20] Create joy and satisfaction. *Mental Health America*. Available from: http://www.mentalhealthamerica.net/create-joy-and-satisfaction. Cited March 7, 2019.

[21] Chang C, Tsai G, Hsieh CJ. Psychological, immunological and physiological effects of a Laughing Qigong Program (LQP) on adolescents. *Complement Ther Med*. 2013 Dec;21(6):660-8. doi: 10.1016/j.ctim.2013.09.004. Epub 2013 Sep 13. PMID: 24280475.

[22] Kim SH, Kook JR, Kwon M, Son MH, Ahn SD, Kim YH. The effects of laughter therapy on mood state and self-esteem in cancer patients undergoing radiation therapy: a randomized controlled trial. *J Altern Complement Med*. 2015 Apr;21(4):217-22. doi: 10.1089/acm.2014.0152. PMID: 25875938.

[23] Heo EH, Kim S, Park HJ, Kil SY. The effects of a simulated laughter programme on mood, cortisol levels, and health-related quality of life among haemodialysis patients. *Complement Ther Clin Pract.* 2016 Nov;25:1-7. doi: 10.1016/j.ctcp.2016.07.001. Epub 2016 Jul 27. PMID: 27863598.

[24] Manninen S, Tuominen L, Dunbar RI, Karjalainen T, Hirvonen J, Arponen E, Hari R, Jääskeläinen IP, Sams M, Nummenmaa L. Social laughter triggers endogenous opioid release in humans. *J Neurosci.* 2017 Jun 21;37(25):6125-6131. doi: 10.1523/ JNEUROSCI.0688-16.2017. Epub 2017 May 23. PMID: 28536272; PMCID: PMC6596504.

[25] Why laughter is good for the immune system, opens inner cellar pharmacy. Available from: https://www. laughteronlineuniversity.com/laughter-immune- system/

[26] Reader's Digest. Available from: https://rd.com/ jokes/knock-knock/